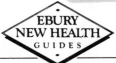

EBURY
NEW HEALTH
G U I D E S

CONTENTS

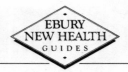

INTRODUCTION

GETTING pregnant is a risky business. In 1983, of more than 89,000 pregnancies in Britain, 27,000 ended in miscarriage, there were 6,000 perinatal deaths, 14,000 babies born with physical defects and 42,000 low birthweight babies. *Roughly one in seven pregnancies go wrong.* And the evidence is that birth defects are on the increase. In 1965, 159 children per thousand births were born with some congenital defect. By 1983, the figure was 221 per thousand. That's the bad news. The good news is that the majority of these problems can be avoided if the mother's nutrition is optimum* prior to, and during, pregnancy.

But even this is only half the story. We believe, from the evidence presented in this book, that if nutrition is better than just adequate, if nutrition is optimum for the individual there are a number of additional benefits. These include: an easier pregnancy, without pregnancy sickness; an easier birth and faster recovery; a larger and healthier baby at birth; a baby more resilient to colds and other childhood ailments; a baby whose mental and physical development reach their full potential and a happier baby that sleeps well at night.

Working with pregnant women over the past five years we have come to the conclusion that the normal experiences of pregnancy, childbirth and early motherhood are far from right. The average birthweight of a baby is around 7½ lb; our clients rarely have a baby under 8 lb. Professor Bryce-Smith, one of Britain's leading investigators into the cause behind miscarriage and malformations, recently concluded that babies born under 6 lb 9 oz should be suspected of sub-optimal nutrition.

The purpose of this book is to give you the evidence to support these claims, but most of all to give you the information for a healthy pregnancy and to make healthy babies.

Optimum nutrition means more than eating a well-balanced diet. It means supplying the ideal level of each nutrient.

EBURY
NEW HEALTH
G U I D E S

THE
BETTER
PREGNANCY
DIET

EBURY PRESS LONDON

L I Z & P A T R I C K H O L F O R D

Published by Ebury Press
Division of the National Magazine Company Ltd
Colquhoun House
27–37 Broadwick Street
London W1V 1FR

ISBN 0 85223 571 2

Edited by Mike Franklin
Designed by Peter Bridgewater Associates
Computerset in Great Britain by
ECM Ltd, London
Printed and bound in Great Britain by
The Bath Press

A complete list of over 100 references, given in the book in brackets, is available from
the Institute of Optimum Nutrition. Please send £1.50 and a SAE to the address at the
back of the book.

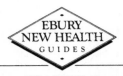
CHAPTER 1

MAXIMUM FERTILITY

THE inability to reproduce is one of the very first signs of less than perfect nutrition. In fact, one of the criteria for deeming a food substance a vitamin and hence essential for life is whether or not it affects fertility.

No less than one in four couples suffer from infertility and the evidence of some researchers suggests even this is a low estimate (1). For some people this means having less children. For most it means having none at all. But even for the fertile couple, getting pregnant isn't as easy as it sounds. The average time it takes to get pregnant is six months, and waiting 18 months is not uncommon. In the absence of fertility tests, infertility is not diagnosed until 18 months have passed.

However, this chapter isn't written just for those who wish to prevent infertility, but also for those parents-to-be who wish to minimize the chance of something going wrong in pregnancy. Concluding their book *Prevention of Handicap and the Health of Women* Arthur and Margaret Wynn stated that in malnutrition epidemics babies were not born to the most ill-fed women, who were infertile, but to the women whose nutrition was marginal so that they were still fertile but not well enough fed to have healthy babies. It has been estimated that only 10 in a hundred people in Britain genuinely receive adequate amounts of all vitamins and minerals to meet the international daily recommendations. You don't just need to be fertile. You need maximum fertility.

WOMEN AREN'T THE ONLY ONES TO BLAME

In the past it has been wrongly assumed that the woman is responsible for the majority of infertile couples, and that birth defects, too, have more to do with the woman. While roughly two-thirds of infertility cases are caused by the woman and one-third by the man (2), defective sperm from the male may cause as much as 80 per cent of birth defects resulting from genetic abnormalities, according to a survey of medical literature in the 1960s by the environmentalist group, Friends of the Earth. Their document stated 'American men presently cause the vast majority of birth defects and sperm counts are the major variable in birth defects.'

There are also degrees of infertility, so a marginally fertile woman married to a man with a low sperm count may not result in conception. Anything that can be done on either side to improve fertility increases the chances of getting pregnant when you want to and also increases your chances for a healthy baby.

Fertility and the speed of conception depend on many factors, some psychological, some physical, some nutritional and some environmental. For example, conceptions are very high during holidays since stress is a major factor in infertility. It is also well known that during food shortages the number of births decline (3). Knowing how to time intercourse to coincide with ovulation (the release of the female egg to be fertilized by the sperm) also greatly increases conception. But most of all, your nutrition, especially your vitamin and mineral status, plays a crucial role.

THE ENDANGERED SPERM

The standard test for fertility for the man is a sperm count which measures number of sperm in a millilitre of semen. Scores of over 100 million are deemed healthy, which is the average sperm count of a fertile man. A sperm count of 90 million or less is found in infertile males. However, it is not only the number of sperm but their motility which determines what chance they have of surviving the 24-hour swim up the fallopian tube, to arrive with enough gusto to deliver their half of the message which begins the life of your baby.

Healthy sperm are in danger of becoming a rare species. In the last 60 years, sperm counts have been dropping substantially. According to some studies, modern man may produce less than a quarter of the sperm compared to the average man 50 years ago. For example, one study by Dr Dougherty at Florida State University found that 23 per cent of the male students had sperm counts of less than 20 million sperm, making them infertile.

This decline in sperm count is probably in part due to increased sex. Abstinence from sex greatly increases sperm concentration. Since today's man has more sex than his counterpart 50 years ago one would expect some decline. However, even with this factor taken into account, sperm counts are decreasing. Why?

Proving why sperm counts are decreasing is no easy task. Even the reliance on sperm count values is criticized. Some researchers devised a method of measuring the motility and ability of sperm to fertilize eggs, using hamster eggs in the laboratory as a target for the sperm under examination. This technique, called the sperm penetration assay, revealed that the sperm of men whose mothers had been treated with the controversial synthetic oestrogen, DES, had impaired ability to penetrate the egg, although their sperm count was unaffected. However, some researchers, like the former Associate Professor of Urology at Washington University, Dr Mark Kiviat, say that this test is 'Hocus pocus. Nobody knows what the test means.' It is likely that a number of drugs affect sperm quantity and quality but proving this is never easy.

Thanks to the Mormons, who avoid coffee, alcohol and cigarettes almost completely, it has been possible to demonstrate a link between these substances and problems of reproduction. For example, there is some evidence that spontaneous abortions, premature births and stillbirths are more common when the father's coffee consumption is high.

THE EFFECTS OF SMOKING

While it is recognized that mothers who smoke run the risk of damaging their babies, the evidence for fathers who smoke is not so clear. If both mother and father smoke, there is a greater risk of having a low birthweight baby than if just the mother smokes. Also, the risk of death in low birthweight babies is increased. However, who knows whether it's the smoking that does it or whether there is some other factor that is different in couples who both smoke?

For smoking in the man to affect the baby either smoking must damage the sperm, resulting in a defective conception, or some chemical present in the semen must be transmitted to the fertilized egg and cause damage that way.

INDUSTRIAL IMPOTENCE

Two chemicals used as fumicides and pesticides, now fortunately banned, have been found to wreak havoc on healthy sperm. These are DBCP and Kepone. In 1973 a company called Life Sciences Products manufactured Kepone without ensuring the proper safety standards to avoid contamination to the plant and the factory workers. By 1975 a number of workers were suffering from headaches and tremors associated with Kepone poisoning. As the evidence emerged showing the extent of the problem not just for employees but for people living nearby the plant, a full investigation was carried out on 100 employees. The investigators found low sperm counts and an unusual proportion of abnormal and non-motile sperm in many of the employees.

Industrial infertility isn't only reserved for historical disasters like these. A recent report by ASTMS funded by the Equal Opportunities Commission called *Reproductive Hazards at Work* outlines some of the industries which are posing serious infertility problems to both men and women at work. These include the textile industry, nurses handling certain anti-cancer drugs and workers exposed to dyes, solvents and weedkillers, and four out of five farmworkers on one Derbyshire farm who independently approached doctors about their impotence.

INCREASING MALE FERTILITY

In practical terms, the first place to start for the man is to avoid coffee, alcohol, cigarettes and exposure to any suspect drugs or industrial chemicals for three months prior to conception. However, total avoidance of environmental chemicals is never possible, so improved nutrition provides an extra degree of protection. Vitamin C, for example, has been shown to protect the smoker from increased blood pressure associated with smoking (4) and may well decrease the risk of sperm damage, too. The importance of vitamin C for increasing fertility has recently been reported in a study by Dr Gonzales (5) which showed that giving extra vitamin C increased sperm count as well as motility. He gave 500 mg of vitamin C twice a day to a group of 35 infertile men and found 'continuous increases in percentage of normal sperm, sperm viability and sperm motility'. The most significant change that occurred to the sperm was a decrease in agglutination (the name given to the clumping together of sperm) which is associated with impaired fertility. The mechanism by which vitamin C increases fertility is not yet known.

Vitamin E deficiency has been found to induce sterility in both sexes by causing damage to the reproductive tissues. Unfortunately, that does not mean that taking vitamin E will reverse sterility (6).

The high rate of infertility in diabetics may provide us with a clue to the role nutrition plays in fertility. Diabetics are also frequently low in vitamin A which is essential for making the male sex hormones. Vitamin A is also dependent on zinc for its release from the liver.

ZINC AND MALE FERTILITY

Of all the nutrients known to affect male fertility, zinc is perhaps the best researched. Signs of zinc deficiency include late sexual maturation, small sex organs and infertility. Zinc deficiency also results in damage to the testes. Short-term zinc deficiency does not result in permanent damage, but long-term deficiency may do.

With adequate supplementation of zinc these problems can be corrected. Dr Pfeiffer, a specialist in mental illness, has also found a high degree of impotence and infertility in his male patients suffering from zinc deficiency (8). 'With adequate dosage of vitamin B6 and zinc, the sexual ability of the male should return in one to two months' time.' In view of the fact that the average dietary intake of zinc has been found to be substantially lower than the intake recommended by the National Research Council (9), the effects of zinc on fertility may be quite substantial. The average intake has been estimated to be as low as 7.9 mg per day, while an intake of 15 mg per day is usually considered appropriate. Zinc is found in high concentrations in the sex glands of the male and also in the sperm itself. There it is needed to make the outer layer and tail and is therefore essential for healthy sperm.

It is still a mystery as to why there is so much zinc in the testes as well as high levels of a particularly complex fatty acid called DHA. Recently it has been suggested that zinc may also be needed to make hormone-like substances in the testes called prostaglandins, which are synthesized from DHA. Supplementing DHA appears, however, to have little effect on the concentration of this fatty acid in the testes (10). The effects of dietary zinc sufficiency or deficiency are much more pronounced. On a zinc-deficient diet the zinc concentration in the testes falls to one-third the normal level (11). As much as 1.4 mg of zinc is lost with each ejaculation, so a prolific sex life and an inadequate diet would put you at risk! In fact, in the nineteenth century many patients were diagnosed as having 'masturbation insanity' – perhaps the earliest suggestion of a link between zinc, sex and mental illness. (There may be more than an element of truth to the old saying that masturbation makes you blind and stunts your growth.)

ZINC AND FEMALE FERTILITY

For women, zinc is also crucial. Problems of fertility, sex drive and menstruation have all been linked to inadequate levels of zinc. The sex hormone gonadotrophin needs zinc and vitamin B6 to be produced in adequate amounts. The beneficial effects of vitamin B6 together with zinc affect every part of the female sexual cycle. They increase desire for sex, alleviate pre-menstrual problems, ease sickness in pregnancy and depression after the birth, as well as increasing the chances of a healthy baby. Essentially, zinc and B6 ensure that adequate levels of sex hormones are produced. For example, one hormone called LHRH (luteinizing hormone releasing hormone) causes the pituitary in the centre of the head to stimulate the development of the ovum and hence ovulation. Deficiency in B6 causes a deficiency in LHRH.

SLIMMING AND INFERTILITY

While it is known that infertility rates go up in times of food shortage, one would have thought that the average person would eat a good enough diet to maintain the ability to reproduce. But according to Swedish information, this is far from the truth. Slimmers run the real risk of stopping their normal menstrual cycle and hence becoming infertile. Of a group of 53 women who became amenorrhoeic due to loss of weight, 25 were purposely on a diet, 10 had psychological problems which had interfered with their eating habits, six were physically ill, four had an insufficient diet, two exercised too much, three did not think they had lost weight and for three the cause was unknown (12).

Advertising perpetuates the myth that all women should conform to the ultra-slim archetype. Some overdo it with serious consequences to health. The Swedish work showed that the weight at which the average woman became amenorrhoeic was 8 st 3 lb for a medium-frame woman. Even the Health Education Council in their booklet *Looking After Yourself* state the 'OK' weight range to be from 7 st 10 lb to 9 st 6 lb.

CHOOSE THE RIGHT METHOD OF CONTRACEPTION

One of the problems with zinc and B6 is not just dietary deficiency, but also the antagonism of the birth control pill. This was discovered when 80 mg of B6 helped those suffering from depression induced by the pill (13). The pill also induces a deficiency of vitamins B and C (14) and especially B12 (15). Since the pill elevates copper levels (16), which has been associated with increased birth defects, one might end up taking 10 vitamin and mineral pills to counteract the dangerous effects of the birth control pill! A much better alternative is to switch to a safer form of contraception, since the use of the pill has also been associated with migraine headaches, cervical cancer and an increase in depression and suicides in young women (17). It is certainly wise to avoid the pill for at least two months before a planned conception.

MAKE LOVE AS NEAR TO OVULATION AS POSSIBLE

Unlike the pill or coil, natural methods of birth control do not interfere with the cycle of ovulation and menstruation. During this cycle, which can vary from 23 to 35 days (18), there is only one day in which the egg is available for fertilization. However, sperms usually live for three days and under excellent conditions can survive for five days. A longer survival rate is extremely rare. Therefore, if one knew when ovulation occurred, abstinence from sex for five days (or the use of a diaphragm or condom) would avoid the chance of pregnancy, while frequent sex would dramatically increase the chance of conception. So, how do you find out when ovulation occurs?

The discovery that a different type of mucus is produced just before ovulation led to the development of the simplest and safest method of birth control. Unlike normal vaginal mucus, fertile mucus is sticky and thread-like mucus, a bit like egg white. This fertile mucus both nourishes and protects the sperm, providing it with channels to move along, thereby greatly increasing its chances of reaching the egg. In a World Health Organization study 90 per cent of women could identify the fertile mucus within the first month. After a little guidance 94 per cent had no problem knowing when ovulation was about to occur. The Billings Method of mucus observation greatly increases one's chance of conception by having sex during the fertile part of the cycle. Details of this simple method of birth control are explained in *The Billings Method* by Dr Billings, published by Allen Lane.

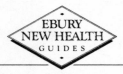

CHAPTER 2

THE POLLUTION-FREE WOMB

THE first nine months of your baby's life are, by all accounts, the most important. During these nine months the baby is totally dependent on nutrition from the mother, receiving nourishment directly into its bloodstream through the placenta. The placenta is the baby's life support system. It consists of a mass of blood vessels which pass food nutrients from your blood down the umbilical cord and into your baby. Spiralling around the umbilicus are blood vessels carrying oxygen to the foetus, and waste materials and carbon dioxide are pumped along two foetal arteries back to the placenta. The placenta also acts as a barrier, preventing all substances in your bloodstream passing directly into the baby. However, it is not a total barrier against drugs, toxic metals, viruses and other undesirables.

Unlike fully grown adults, the unborn baby is highly sensitive to the slightest changes in the supply of nutrients or indeed poisons. So much so that the mother may be perfectly healthy yet pass on dangerous deficiencies or excesses to the unborn child. For instance, low folic acid levels in mothers have been shown to be probably the most significant factor in spina bifida babies, whose neural tubes don't develop properly, resulting in severe disability. Yet the marginally folic acid deficient mother may show no signs of deficiency.

ANTI-NUTRIENTS IN PREGNANCY

More than any other time in one's life, nutrition needs to be optimum, not just adequate, if you want a truly healthy baby. But good nutrition isn't just about what you eat, it's also about what you don't eat, drink or breathe. Many of the substances considered to be bad for us, like alcohol, lead fumes and cigarettes, cause their damage by interfering with essential nutrients. For instance, lead is a powerful antagonist to zinc and to calcium, both crucial for mental and physical development. These anti-nutrients, perhaps harmless for adults in tiny quantities, can be dangerous for the baby.

But in a world where each one of us on average eats 14 pounds of preservatives and additives, breathes one gram of heavy metals and has one gallon of pesticides and herbicides sprayed on our healthy fruit and vegetables each year, it is hard to distinguish between what is normal mental and physical development in a baby and what should be normal. Only when the effects of anti-nutrients like lead pollution or drugs like Thalidomide become so gross do we do anything about it.

LEAD AND PREGNANCY

In 1980, Professor Bryce-Smith at the University of Reading set out to see whether birth abnormalities or miscarriages had anything to do with the mother's mineral levels. His results, discussed more fully in Chapter 5, have clearly shown a direct relationship between lead levels in the placenta and the birthweight of the baby. Perhaps more interesting is the fact that this correlation exists even in mothers whose lead levels would be considered normal. Like many environmental poisons, there appears to be no threshold at which lead could be categorically called safe.

Further evidence for the dangers of low-level lead have recently been reported by child psychiatrist Professor Herbert Needleman. He found that lead levels recorded at birth correlate with intellectual development at age three. That lead has emerged as a factor in the birthweight and intelligence of children further confirms the notion that known toxins may show effects at doses considered safe in foetal development.

However, these are the effects of levels of lead common to all of us. What of the small percentage that are exposed to higher lead intakes? From what is known about lead one would expect it to damage sperm and ova, and indeed it does. Levels of 0.3 parts per million in animals are enough to cause foetal damage. That's not so much higher than our average level in Britain of around 0.1 ppm. (Manchester, our most polluted city, has a lead level of 0.17 ppm on average.) When intakes of the essential minerals calcium, zinc or iron are low, lead becomes that much more toxic. Given that many pregnant women are deficient in all three, caution is required. After all, there is already some evidence that stillborn babies or aborted foetuses have higher lead levels than average (1). Like the canaries used to detect gas in coal mines in days of old, the unborn baby sadly serves as our most sensitive early warning system for the ravages of world pollution.

COPPER AND PREGNANCY

Copper is both an essential element and a toxic one. Due to the widespread use of copper in water pipes, jewellery, kitchen utensils, IUDs, swimming pool anti-fungal agents and coins modern man is more at risk from toxicity than deficiency. Of the 2 mg we need each day, that amount is supplied simply from drinking water that has passed through copper pipes, irrespective of any copper that is absorbed from our food.

Copper levels in the blood tend to rise dramatically during pregnancy and remain elevated for five weeks after birth (2). It is thought that copper may act as a stimulus for the uterus and therefore be necessary in pregnancy. Because of its natural increase in pregnancy, copper toxicity is far more common during pregnancy than at other times. Too much too soon may be a factor in inducing premature babies or miscarriages.

High levels of copper may also be a factor in inducing post-natal depression or mental illness. Copper depresses histamine levels in the body and since histamine is an important nerve transmitter this in turn affects the brain. The signs of copper toxicity include hypertension and mental illness.

Copper is very antagonistic to zinc and therefore extra zinc, as well as vitamin C, can help to detoxify copper. A balance of 14 parts of zinc to every one part of copper is needed to provide some protection against copper toxicity. Yet many supplements contain 2 mg of copper and 5 mg of zinc. To be balanced such a formula should contain 28 mg of zinc. Copper levels can be determined simply by hair mineral analysis. Unless the hair is permed this is a good provisional test for copper status.

MERCURY AND PREGNANCY

The saying 'mad as a hatter' originated because hatters used to polish top hats with mercury. And mercury, like lead, is extremely toxic. In elevated amounts it is highly teratogenic (literally, 'monster-producing'). In the Minimata Bay disaster in Japan (1953–60) 111 people died and many more children were born disabled after eating fish contaminated with mercury from a local plastics factory. In some fish caught in polluted waters (and that would certainly include the English Channel and, for most of Britain, most coastal waters) mercury levels are high. Our other common source of mercury is dental fillings.

However, unlike lead and copper it is not commonly available and as such it is rare to find individuals who are mercury toxic.

According to Professor Bryce-Smith 'Exposure to mercury does increase allergic sensitivity and it is likely that one per cent, or at most five per cent, of people may react to mercury fillings.' The mercury in teeth is not totally immobile and it is possible to detect traces of mercury in the breath of people with mercury fillings. After fillings have been fitted or removed, urinary mercury also may show a slight increase, although this soon disappears. Although the danger from mercury fillings is really of a very small magnitude it is a wise precaution not to have dental work involving fitting or removing mercury fillings during pregnancy.

PROTECT YOURSELF FROM POLLUTION

Toxic minerals are in the air, the soil and food. Over the past 100 years, their levels have risen sharply, and could well be overloading the body's capacity to eliminate them. Here's what to do to keep your exposure to the minimum.

- Avoid busy roads where possible. Exhaust fumes contain lead.
- Wash all fruit and vegetables.
- Remove outer leaves of vegetables.
- Wash hands before eating.
- Make sure small children don't chew on paintwork.
- Avoid copper or aluminium cookware.
- Don't wrap food in aluminium foil.
- Avoid canned goods, which may be contaminated with aluminium or lead.
- Cut down on alcohol, which increases lead absorption.
- Avoid antacids which contain aluminium salts.
- Avoid refined foods, which lack toxin-fighting nutrients.
- Check if your water pipes are made of lead or copper. If so don't use a water softener. Soft water dissolves lead more easily; do not drink or cook with hot tap water; use a water filter or drink distilled or spring water.

DETOXIFY YOUR BODY

It isn't possible to avoid the full extent of pollution. Luckily, research is showing that there are ways of detoxifying the body. Drugs are effective, but cause side effects; a safer and equally effective way is to ensure a carefully balanced nutrition.

THE DETOXIFYING DIET

◆ Calcium and phosphorus are antagonistic to lead. They are found in seeds, nuts, green leafy vegetables and milk produce.

◆ Alginic acid is also a lead antagonist. It is found in seaweed (provided it comes from unpolluted waters). If seaweed sounds unappetising, try Nori. This comes in dried sheets which are crisped by heating them without oil in a very hot pan for less than 10 seconds, and then used as a crunchy garnish for soups and salads.

◆ Pectin helps remove lead too. It is found in apple pips, bananas, citrus fruit and carrots.

◆ Sulphur-containing amino acids, which are found in garlic, onions and eggs, help protect against mercury, cadmium and lead.

SUPPLEMENTS AGAINST POLLUTION

Hair mineral analysis is an accurate way to measure body levels of these toxins. Where body levels of toxins are too high, diet alone cannot supply nutritional antagonists in doses high enough to be effective. Several research projects have shown, however, that certain nutrients are very effective in supplement form.

◆ Vitamin C is an 'all rounder' which escorts lead, cadmium and arsenic out of the body.

◆ Calcium is effective against lead, cadmium and aluminium.

◆ Zinc acts against lead and cadmium.

◆ Selenium is antagonistic to mercury and, to a lesser extent, arsenic and cadmium.

◆ Pectin, alginic acid and phosphorus are also useful as supplements.

◆ Magnesium and B6 are useful for detoxifying aluminium.

THE DRUGS TO AVOID BEFORE
AND DURING PREGNANCY

Any drug treatment is to be avoided if at all possible during pregnancy. According to Dr Scott, an obstetrician and former member of the British Committee on Safety of Medicines, 'Practitioners must be taught and retaught that drug therapy should only be used in pregnancy for the most pressing indicators.' Most drugs are never tested in clinical trials on pregnant women for obvious ethical reasons. Therefore, it is often not known how the unborn child may react.

Most drugs are low in molecular weight and pass easily through the placenta into the foetus. The Thalidomide disaster debunked once and for all the idea that the placenta protects the foetus from drugs taken by the mother. However, most people put drugs like this in a totally different category from sleeping pills, pain killers or tranquillizers. Although these common drugs do not cause toxic disasters as witnessed by Thalidomide, they are still toxic substances which the unborn child is not designed to cope with and they should be avoided where possible. Even a single aspirin has been reported in one man to have caused intestinal bleeding for a week! (3)

Sleeping Tablets, Antibiotics and Tranquillizers

Sleeping tablets, antibiotics and tranquillizers have been tentatively linked to a greater risk of childhood cancer. The Oxford Survey for Childhood Cancer have been collecting information on every child who has died of cancer in Britain since the 1950s. During the period 1972–77 there was a statistically greater risk of a child dying of cancer if the mother had used these drugs during pregnancy. In the case of antibiotics it isn't known whether it was the drug or the virus for which the antibiotic was prescribed that was at fault. Childhood cancer is fortunately very rare. There is a less than one in a thousand chance of a child dying of cancer. Of the few who do, possibly a quarter are in part caused by drugs during pregnancy. Sedative drugs like phenobarbitone are to be avoided at all costs.

Aspirin

Even the most common drug of all, aspirin, is associated with decreased birthweight. In a survey in Scotland, an average 54 per cent of women used aspirin (salicylic acid) for a total of 31 days during pregnancy (4). In the laboratory, aspirin has been shown to reduce rates of DNA synthesis, and suppress immune function, which are the markers of a drug that can affect foetal development. While there is no conclusive proof that aspirins are harmful in pregnancy, they have been shown in studies on rats to result in lower birthweight (5).

The Pill

The birth control pill is another drug which depresses immune function. According to Dr Peebles, it is 'sensible to allow two or three menstrual cycles to pass between stopping an oral contraceptive regime and starting a pregnancy. Even disregarding other notable effects, it is a good idea to establish a regular cycle before conception.'

Cannabis

Cannabis is a recreational drug that suppresses immune function. Although not in the same league as Thalidomide, cannabis and other immune-suppressant drugs have been shown to greatly reduce the number of brain cells in young animals. Whether this effect occurs in humans is not established.

REDUCING THE TOXICITY OF DRUGS WITH NUTRIENTS

It is inevitable that some pregnant women may need to be prescribed a drug during pregnancy. The potential danger of drugs can be reduced by ensuring nutrition is optimum. Even drugs like Thalidomide were found to become more toxic if vitamin deficiency existed. Deficiencies of vitamin A, B2, pantothenic acid (B5), folic acid, B12 and vitamin E all increased the risk of birth defects with Thalidomide. In the words of the Swiss physician Paracelsus, 'Only the dose makes the poison,' and vitamin deficiency effectively lowers the dose that can be tolerated without ill effect.

NITRATES AND CANCER

Professor Knox at Birmingham University said 'Pregnant rats given very small doses of certain chemicals called nitrosamines develop cancer in a very predictable way.' Nitrosamines are very potent carcinogens (cancer-producing agents). They are formed either in food or during digestion from the combination of nitrates or nitrites and amines, which are protein-particles. Every year, farmers add tons of nitrate-nitrogen compounds on to the soil to encourage the plants to grow faster. Nitrogen is a vital constituent of protein and thus allows the plants to be more productive. But if these compounds are not used up by the plant during growth, they will accumulate nitrates and pass these on to whoever eats them. Nitrates can change to nitrites, and nitrites to nitrosamines, the carcinogenic compound. Nitrates are also used in many meat products as preservatives. Almost all pies, sausages, hamburgers and processed meats are rich in nitrates. Obviously avoiding all nitrates is impractical, so what can you do?

Firstly, avoid processed meats containing additives E250, E251 or

E252. If you're lucky enough to have access to organically grown fruit and vegetables, all the better; or grow your own without artificial fertilizers. Finally, take plenty of vitamin C because this prevents the conversion of nitrites and amines to form nitrosamines.

THE GREEN POTATO POISON

The active poison known for years to be present in green potatoes has been identified as alpha-solanine and alpha-chaconine. These are known to cause spina bifida in animals. The strange finding that spina bifida incidence was concentrated in certain areas and was particularly high in Ireland may be due to eating large amounts of potatoes. In 1973 a report showed seasonal patterns of spina bifida and was associated with the sprouting of potatoes in the spring, while a 1966 report correlated periods of potato blight with increased incidence of neural tube defect (7). Be extra careful not to eat the green bits when you're pregnant!

IS COFFEE BAD FOR YOU?

Research on caffeine in coffee has recently clearly established the potential of this common drink to be carcinogenic, at least in large quantities. But can it damage the unborn child? According to a survey from Finland, where more coffee is drunk than anywhere else in the world, there is no greater risk for birth abnormalities in coffee drinkers (8). However, results of two new animal studies confirm earlier reports that caffeine is a teratogen when administered to pregnant animals at high doses. Minimum doses required are 100 mg/kg body weight, which is way beyond the amounts one would get from drinking coffee (9). However, you may wish to try tasty alternatives like dandelion coffee or herb teas.

While all the 'anti-nutrients' covered in this chapter are bad for you and your baby in large quantities it is really the overall exposure to such pollutants that makes the difference. Many poisons store in fatty tissue and over the years can become increasingly toxic. By doing your best to reduce your overall body burden of pollutants you provide your baby with the healthiest environment in which to thrive and grow in its first nine months of life.

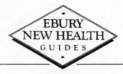

CHAPTER 3

THE DANGERS OF DRINKING AND SMOKING

TODAY, more than ever before, miscarriage is the greatest threat to any pregnancy. One in 10 pregnancies ends in miscarriage. This figure is likely to be an underestimate since early miscarriages are often not reported and often go unnoticed. It has been estimated that for every successful conception there are three early miscarriages in which the ovum may have been fertilized but failed to implant properly. The woman may notice nothing more than a delayed or missed period, sometimes followed by a heavier period than usual. Once a pregnancy is beyond 28 weeks, one in every 65 women will lose her baby (1).

Experts believe that miscarriage is the most sensitive of all indications that a woman or her partner are exposed to environmental hazards (2). Researchers from Columbia University in New York decided to investigate the risk factors associated with miscarriage in 2,802 New York women. They found that the risk of miscarriage increased with consumption of cigarettes and alcohol. A drinker and smoker had a four times higher risk of miscarriage. Those who didn't smoke but had a drink every day still had a risk more than 2.5 times higher than the abstainer.

ALCOHOL AND MISCARRIAGE

Certainly the most wide-spread poison for the unborn child is alcohol. Although there has been a flurry of concern and research in the last decade confirming the potentially damaging effects of even small quantities of alcohol during pregnancy, the concept at least is nothing new.

More than 3,000 years ago a messenger from God warned Samson's mother, in the Bible, Judges 13, 'You are going to conceive and have a son. Now see to it that you drink no wine or other fermented drink.' In Carthage and Sparta newly-weds were banned from drinking alcohol to prevent 'conception during intoxication'. Some 250 years ahead of his time, Dr James Sedgewick published in a *Treatise on Liquors* 'the train of chronic diseases with which we see children afflicted (were) brought on infants by the debauchery of the mother . . . so that, from the whole, the regulation of the mother during pregnancy is an affair of the highest moment and consideration'. But not until 1981, in a landmark report in the *International Journal of Environmental Studies*, were these suspicions once and for all confirmed by Mrs Holland, the chairman of the National Council of Women Working Party on Alcohol Problems, concluding that 'alcohol is the third most common environmental cause of difficulties in the development of an unborn child' (3). Let's examine the evidence.

THE FETAL ALCOHOL SYNDROME

Miscarriage may be nature's way of terminating a pregnancy that was destined to go wrong, but many babies are born suffering from the effects of maternal alcohol consumption. The signs and symptoms, now well documented, are known as fetal alcohol syndrome. 'Its main signs are low birthweight and mild facial deformity', according to a report in the *New Scientist* in August 1985. 'The flattened midface, often with a thin upper lip, is connected to a short nose with little nostril flare. The eyelid openings are short, the ears often misshapen, and the lower jaw long. Many affected babies also have heart murmurs, persistent ear infections leading to deafness, droopy eyelids, squint, congenital hip dislocations, and fingers and toes that may be short, partly fused, angled, lacking in flexion, and with small nails.' These are the most common physical abnormalities resulting from alcohol in pregnancy.

Alcohol also affects mental development and behaviour too. Victims of fetal alcohol syndrome are often hyperactive, jittery and have difficulty sleeping. But a baby doesn't have to have the physical signs to be mentally defected by alcohol, according to Canadian researchers at Queens University in Ontario. They investigated whether there was any difference in mental development in children whose mothers drank or smoked at socially accepted levels during pregnancy. They found that verbal skills, both in speaking and understanding, were poorer in the children from these mothers (4).

HOW MUCH IS TOO MUCH?

Nobody really knows how much is too much and while a report by the Royal College of Psychiatrists in London stated that 'a couple of bottles of wine taken each day is getting into the danger area' (5), Dr Woollam, the consultant to the World Health Organization, with 25 years of research into environmental hazards including Thalidomide, says 'No alcohol during pregnancy is the only safe limit.' His views are backed up by the recent Columbia University study which showed that even the consumption of a single drink every other day increased the risk of miscarriage.

Professor David Smith from Washington, recognized as a world authority on fetal alcohol syndrome, points out that 'there is no known teratogen yet studied in man which clearly shows a threshold effect where the substance is quite safe to a particular level, beyond which it is teratogenic'.

Many environmental hazards, including alcohol, are at their most dangerous at the very early stages of pregnancy, when cell division is at its highest. So alcohol really needs to be avoided from the time a couple chooses to get pregnant, not just when the woman discovers she is. While the first 20 weeks are deemed the most critical stage during which alcohol should be avoided, Dr Ann Streissguth, who was one of the first doctors to identify the characteristics of fetal alcohol syndrome, says that 'experiments on animals demonstrate that babies exposed to alcohol only in the later stages of pregnancy are still susceptible to behavioural problems' (6). While it had been hoped that children would grow out of these physical and mental defects, it is now clear that they don't. In a follow-up study on 10 fetal alcohol syndrome children by Ann Streissguth, two are dead, and the rest are backward or subnormal.

But it isn't only the woman who needs to abstain. Alcohol damages sperm, and at least in animals, alcohol consumption in the male does result in a greater risk for birth defects and miscarriage in future children (7). So save the champagne till after the birth, and even then don't have too much if you're breast feeding!

ALCOHOL RAISES YOUR BLOOD PRESSURE

Women with a history of moderately high blood pressure would do well to avoid alcohol at any time but especially during pregnancy. Alcohol has been found to be a major factor contributing to raised blood pressure, which over 10 per cent of all women suffer from. Being overweight is, of course, another major factor (9). And once again, you don't have to drink a lot to be affected according to one, no doubt popular, group of researchers. They gave patients entering hospital a can of beer a day to investigate whether the slight decrease in blood pressure during short stays in hospital was due to reduction in alcohol consumption. Sure enough, on their can of beer a day, blood pressure no longer declined during their stay.

ALCOHOL THE ANTI-NUTRIENT

Alcohol is the best example of a substance that may do its damage by compromising good nutrition. As well as affecting absorption of nutrients, it interferes with their positive health action in body chemistry. Nutrients like B6, iron and zinc, so badly needed during pregnancy, are badly affected when alcohol is drunk in excess. This leads to greater needs for B6 which are higher anyway during pregnancy.

Most of all, alcohol consumption badly affects the availability of zinc, so crucial for pregnancy. Research at Oregon State University has revealed that consumption of alcohol while on a zinc-sufficient diet produces zinc deficiency equivalent to that of a zinc-deficient diet without any extra alcohol. So alcohol is a powerful anti-zinc factor during gestation and lactation (10).

HOW WIDESPREAD IS THE ALCOHOL PROBLEM?

It is likely that the dangers of alcohol in pregnancy will become increasingly apparent, due to the ever-increasing incidence of alcoholism in women. In 1966 there was only one female alcoholic to every eight men. By 1979 it was one to one. Now for every man with a drinking problem there are two women. In Britain alone there are over a million women addicted to alcohol and many more who are socially dependent.

CIGARETTES AND PREGNANCY

Every year, more than 500 medical papers are published on smoking. It is now clear that smoking in pregnancy reduces birthweight, affects mental development of the child in later years and provides an increased risk of cancer to both mother and baby.

The Royal College of Physicians' report *Health or Smoking* concludes 'Women who smoke are more likely to be infertile or take longer to conceive than women who do not smoke. Smokers who become pregnant have a small increase in the risk of spontaneous abortion, bleeding during pregnancy and the development of various placental abnormalities.' But most marked of all is the incidence of low birth-weight babies among smoking mothers.

SMOKING REDUCES GROWTH RATE OF THE FOETUS

This effect on birth size is caused by cigarette smoke's ability to slow down the rate of growth of the foetus. It may do this by damaging the DNA, our blueprint for survival. This in turn has far more serious consequences for mental and physical development. These consequences include a greater risk of having a premature baby, a reduced ability to ward off infection for the young infant and lower mental development (11).

In a study in which women were divided into expected weight of offspring, then either given multivitamin supplements or not, there was a significant difference in weight of baby between those who smoked more than 10 cigarettes a day and were supplemented and those who smoked and were not. The supplementation appeared to offer some protection against the risk of low birthweight (12).

SMOKING LOWERS INTELLIGENCE

The effects of maternal smoking can be seen many years later in the child. A massive survey at Pennsylvania State University involving 9,024 children looked at differences between children who were born to mothers who smoked during pregnancy compared to children of the same mothers when the mother didn't smoke during the pregnancy. 'This study confirms reports that children of women who smoked cigarettes throughout pregnancy have small impairments in intelligence and increased frequencies of short attention span and hyperactive behaviour.' (13)

SMOKING INCREASES ILLNESSES IN CHILDREN

An important concept in nutrition today is that of 'organ reserve'. It's like being born with £100 in the bank. As each organ is taxed the bank balance drops. Eventually the organ will malfunction, but before that, the reserve that organ has may already have diminished substantially. People with low organ reserve may function fine until their body is subjected to stress. Those with weak immune systems are more susceptible to infections, those with poor hormone and nerve balance succumb to the ravages of stress. Children born to mothers who smoke appear to have an overall poor organ reserve, as illustrated by their greater susceptibility to illness. Dr Rantakallio compared frequency of illness in children of smokers or non-smokers and found a 43 per cent increase in illnesses among the smokers' children. These included more blood disorders, more nervous system and sense disorders, more respiratory infections, more bladder and kidney problems and more skin disorders.

HOW TO STOP SMOKING

By now you have probably got the message that smoking during pregnancy is bad news indeed. But what can you do to stop? For the hardened smoker simple words of advice are not enough. Support is needed to kick this habit and a number of organizations exist to provide this. The best course I know for stopping smoking is called Habit Breakers. Their course consists of seven evening sessions, during the first five of which you can smoke. There are no gimmicks, no hypnotism, acupuncture or herbal remedies – most of which have, at most, a few anecdotal reports of success. Habit Breakers have a documented success rate of 69 per cent for people one year after the course.

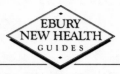

CHAPTER 4

MINIMIZING THE RISK OF BIRTH DEFECTS

O NE in 60 babies is born with some form of mental or physical defect. Most of these tragedies could have been avoided if the parents had known what to do. Although nobody ever believes that it will happen to them, it's as well to understand what these problems are and minimize the risk of anything going wrong.

The growing foetus is most at risk during the first six weeks of pregnancy. During this time the cells divide more frequently. Nutritional inadequacy is known to be able to slow down cell division and the consequences of this in early pregnancy are far more significant. Cell division is like doubling numbers – 2, 4, 8, 16, 32, 64, 128 and so on. Leave out one and the reduction in the total number of cells at birth can be appreciable. It has been calculated that the effects of a cell not doubling in early pregnancy can be the difference between a 3,500 g baby and a 2,500 g baby.

Given that most women don't even discover that they are pregnant till one month after the event, optimum nutrition must start pre-conceptually if the risk of birth defects is to be minimized.

PREVENTING BIRTH ABNORMALITIES

A crucial mineral found to be involved in preventing birth abnormalities is manganese. In a study from Istanbul the concentration of manganese in human hair was measured in mothers and babies. Babies who were born with congenital malformations were significantly lower in hair manganese, as were their mothers. This suggests that manganese deficiency may be another cause for birth abnormalities (3). Manganese is particularly low in cow's milk and also in breast milk of manganese-deficient mothers. Absorption as well as supply is crucial for manganese. Some individuals absorb as little as 2 per cent of the manganese present in diet (4).

Another crucial mineral is zinc. Researchers at the University of

California have shown that zinc deficiency in pregnant rats will result in many stillborn young, and that those born may have one of a number of defects (5). The role of zinc is discussed fully in the next chapter.

SPINA BIFIDA – A FOLIC ACID DEFICIENCY DISEASE?

The two B vitamins folic acid and B12 are both essential for making DNA and RNA and for making normal red blood cells and bone marrow (the base material for cells of the immune system). Folic acid deficiency was first noted in pregnancy in 1945 by Dr Tom Spies, as causing a type of anaemia which went away with folic acid supplementation.

In 1980 Dr Smithells showed in a study of mothers with a high risk of spina bifida babies that only one out of 178 babies had spina bifida in those who took a multivitamin supplement, compared to 23 out of 260 who weren't given the supplement.

The Department of Health and Social Security responded to the importance of this work and the Medical Research Council was called in to fund a large trial to test the effects of supplementation in 4,000 mothers at risk. However, the trial involved some women taking placebo tablets not containing folic acid and there was a public outcry among many medical researchers who believed the trial was unethical because some women with a known risk would be deprived of folic acid although enough evidence already existed to confirm the link between folic acid deficiency and spina bifida.

A recent study by the DHSS supports the importance of folic acid not only in pregnancy, but before pregnancy. In a study which investigated the link between certain drugs and birth defects, it was revealed that mothers who were supplementing folic acid before pregnancy had a lower incidence of spina bifida (8).

Folic acid in food is easily destroyed by sunlight, heat or an acid environment. Much of the folic acid in food can be lost at room temperature or by cooking. Folic acid is thought to be manufactured to some extent by the bacteria in the intestinal tract. Overuse of antibiotics may therefore be another factor promoting deficiency.

According to the World Health Organization one-third to one-half of expectant mothers suffer folic acid deficiency in the last three months of pregnancy (9). The recommended daily allowance in America is between 400 and 500 mcg a day and 800 mcg for a pregnant woman. In Britain the average daily intake is less than 200 mcg. The foetus draws on the mother's folic acid for its own growth, and deficiency is therefore more common in pregnancy. However, insufficient supply for the growing baby may not result in any signs of deficiency in the mother, so supplementation is the only way of ensuring you get enough. According to Dr Pfeiffer, 'Many women with histories of abortion and miscarriage have been able to complete successful childbirth subsequent to folic acid supplementation.'

The drug Valproic acid used for the treatment of epilepsy may also cause spina bifida, according to a letter in the *Lancet*. This drug should also be avoided before or during pregnancy (10).

DOWN'S SYNDROME

When researcher Dr Ruth Harrell heard of a case history reported by biochemist Mary Allen in which the IQ of a Down's Syndrome child went from 20 to 90 points, she decided she had to test the idea that mentally retarded children, even those with genetic defects like Down's Syndrome, may benefit from optimum nutrition. In her study she took 22 mentally retarded children and divided them into two groups. One received supplements containing large amounts of vitamins and minerals. The other group received dummy tablets. The group taking the supplements had an increase of between 5 and 9.6 IQ points; those on dummy tablets showed no change. For the next four months both groups of children were given the supplements and the average improvement was 10.2 points. Six of the Down's Syndrome children had improvements of between 10 and 25 IQ points! The results seemed too good to be true, since this improvement would put most educationally sub-normal children back in normal classes.

Since Ruth Harrell's famous trial, some studies have confirmed her results, while others have not. One replicate study using the same protocol as Harrell's found no significant change in the intelligence of Down's Syndrome children (11). One possible reason could relate to the Down's Syndrome children often needing thyroid drugs to stimulate the thyroid gland. A more recent investigation into Dr Harrell's findings did show that those children on thyroid medication and multivitamins got better. In this replicate study, one Down's Syndrome child was identified as low thyroid and through thyroid medication had a seven-point increase in IQ. Supplements alone did not appear to work (12). Perhaps it is the combination of thyroid hormone plus nutrients that made the difference.

MENTAL RETARDATION

The brain is the most complicated part of any human being and as such is the most vulnerable. This mere 2 lb of delicate software uses up almost half the energy derived from food when a person is at rest. In the growing foetus, the nerve cells in the brain called neurons are rapidly made and by week 20 the unborn child has as many neurons as an adult. Then the wiring begins. Each neuron must interconnect with other neurons by sending out branches. This process is called arborization. Each neuron connects up with approximately 10,000 other neurons, forming a remarkably complex and integral web. This is the centre of our intelligence. The process of arborization still remains a mystery to scientists. Involving both our genetic instructions contained in DNA and feedback through the senses, a new-born baby rapidly develops an intelligence far beyond that of any other living animal.

Arborization happens towards the end of pregnancy and continues throughout childhood, especially in the early stages of a baby's life. It is assumed, although it is impossible to test for obvious moral and ethical reasons, that nutrition plays a major role in brain development. Zinc, for example, promotes DNA production, and zinc antagonists like lead are known, from research, to stunt arborization by up to 10 per cent in animals.

What we do know about nutrition and brain development is that in small-for-date babies there are definite signs of mental retardation, manifesting as poor co-ordination and slow reaction to stimuli (13). Animals born to zinc-deficient mothers show slow learning and more aggressive behaviour towards unpleasant stimuli (14,15). A survey of mentally retarded patients in Finland revealed that 'a remarkably large number of cases have primary cerebral maldevelopment suggesting a pre-natal origin' (16). Small head circumference at birth is therefore of primary importance, and Professor Bryce-Smith's work suggests that nutrition plays a critical role.

More tenuous is the connection between low birthweight or poor physical growth and intelligence. However, it does appear even here that despite different environments for learning, the intelligence of a child at age six is more likely to be high if birthweight was high. Two groups of children in Detroit were divided into high IQ (average 121) and low IQ (average 70). The difference in birthweight was 3,750 g for the high IQ children, compared to 3,020 g for the others (17).

COT DEATHS – A NUTRITION CONNECTION?

Canadian researchers have discovered a clue to the mystery of cot deaths. Cot-death babies have a strikingly greater concentration of dopamine in their carotid glands. These glands regulate breathing and the oxygen balance. Too much dopamine could suppress these and cause death. The conversion of dopamine into the hormone adrenalin is dependent on copper. The roles of copper and its antagonist zinc have yet to be explored.

Deficiency of vitamin A and toxicity of iron has also been implicated in cot deaths. Too much iron can cause extra oxidation of fat-soluble vitamins like vitamin A, so some researchers thought that excessive iron in pregnancy, coupled with low vitamin A levels, might result in liver failure. This avenue has not however proven to provide an explanation for cot deaths (18).

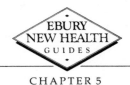

CHAPTER 5

ZINC BABIES THINK BIG

W HY are some babies bigger than others? Is it the diet? Is it genetic? Or is it . . . zinc? The importance of zinc in pre-natal and post-natal health, both for mum and baby, is nothing new. Zinc is involved in about 100 different enzyme reactions in the body, many of which are involved in growth. And it is during times of greatest growth (pregnancy, puberty, wound healing) that zinc deficiency can wreak havoc. In fact, zinc deficiency is associated with genetic abnormalities, because DNA and RNA, which hold the 'blueprint' for our cells, can't function without zinc. Low levels of zinc are found in stillborn babies and even potential fathers become infertile without it.

But what is new and vitally important is the startling research findings of Professor Bryce-Smith on so-called 'normal' mothers and babies.

WHAT IS NORMAL?

After some initial discoveries that high lead and cadmium levels and low zinc were associated with stillbirths, difficult pregnancies and deformed babies, it was imperative to launch a comprehensive study to determine just how important these minerals are. So in 1980 Professor Bryce-Smith set out to test no less than 36 different minerals in a dozen different ways, both in mums and babies. He measured hair levels, blood levels, amniotic fluid, placental levels, pubic hair, cord blood . . . you name it, he tested it! The first question he asked was 'What is normal?' and to find this out he selected 100 normal births, producing normal babies. Much to his surprise, their mineral levels were far from normal. He found that the lower the zinc levels in the placenta, the smaller the baby, and the higher the lead and cadmium levels, the smaller the baby. So clear were the results that Professor Bryce-Smith can predict both birthweight and head circumference just from analyzing these minerals in the placenta! He also found a tendency for high aluminium levels in those who had premature membrane rupture. Iron, the old favourite, had no effect on birth-weight or ease of birth, although there was some evidence of low iron levels in some of the mothers.

When it is considered that these are results of research into 'normal' births, one wonders what will be found in his later research into miscarriages and birth defects (170 tested so far). Dr Golub and workers in California concluded after years of research into zinc that inadequate dietary zinc during pregnancy can lead to restriction of foetal growth, higher than normal incidence of delivery complications, and puts children at a disadvantage during subsequent periods of rapid growth (1). As far as Professor Bryce-Smith is concerned, the link between zinc and birthweight is so strong that he believes that any baby born under 3,000 g (6 lb 9 oz) should immediately be suspected of zinc deficiency. And that's a lot of babies, from a lot of zinc-deficient mums. So why are we all so zinc deficient?

Firstly, according to the US National Academy of Sciences, a pregnant woman needs 20 mg of zinc a day, and 25 mg when breast feeding. In Britain, the average daily intake is 10.5 mg and even less for vegetarians. The sad truth is that even if your diet is exceptionally good, it's nearly impossible to get enough zinc. Consequently, researchers have measured declining levels of zinc in the plasma of pregnant mothers. In first-time mothers with a risk for growth-retarded babies due to their own low weight increase during pregnancy, zinc plasma levels are significantly lower (2).

One of the reasons for zinc deficiency is the worldwide use of phosphate fertilizers. These phosphates stop the plant from absorbing zinc from the soil. One way round this is to eat organic foods.

The foods that are highest in zinc are protein-forming foods. Meat and fish are therefore good sources, but Professor Bryce-Smith warns against fish from polluted waters for pregnant women because of the high cadmium and lead levels. The effect of pollution on fish is critical as illustrated in studies in America, in which the fish from five polluted rivers were examined. No less than 30 per cent of the fish in two of the rivers had cancer – and all the fish in one river had liver cancer!

COPPER VERSUS ZINC

Another way of increasing zinc absorption is to check for copper excess. Copper is a zinc antagonist and Professor Bryce-Smith's research has shown that too much copper and too little zinc again relates to low birthweight. He reported that there was no evidence that copper supplementation is required during pregnancy. However, of the two in a thousand babies born over 4,500 g (9 lb 9 oz) both high zinc and copper are found. So when zinc status is more than adequate, a little extra copper may not be detrimental. The danger is that we can easily get excess copper from environmental exposure to water passing through copper pipes, copper pots and pans and even copper IUDs. No similar environmental sources exist for zinc.

TOO MUCH IRON DEPLETES ZINC

There is also a growing feeling that the traditional iron supplementation of 75.6 mg (in Pregnavite Forte tablets, for example) is far too high as too much iron can also deplete zinc. Provided there is no evidence of iron-deficiency anaemia, 18 mg a day is usually more than enough. After all, the cessation of menstruation means iron is better conserved during pregnancy, menstruation being a major reason for low iron status in women.

It has been suggested that excess iron is a detrimental factor since iron inhibits zinc absorption. Some researchers decided to test whether supplementing iron to a group of marginally zinc-deficient animals would further reduce the birthweight of the offspring, but the results were negative. The extra iron didn't affect the birthweight, nor did it produce a significant change in zinc levels in the offspring. Zinc supplementation, on the other hand, had a significant effect on birthweight, confirming Professor Bryce-Smith's findings (3). During pregnancy, especially towards the end, zinc absorption is very high. Premature infants fed zinc also show greatly increased zinc absorption of 60 per cent (4).

ORANGES HELP ABSORB ZINC

Although oranges may not always contain much vitamin C, they do contain citric acid, which has been positively identified as a factor for increasing absorption of zinc. This is why zinc in breast milk is much better absorbed than zinc in cow's milk because of the citrate content. Colostrum, the first type of breast milk produced immediately after the birth, is particularly high in zinc as well as other nutrients. Colostrum is of vital importance in giving the baby a good start in life after the traumas of the birth. Perhaps this is Nature's way of making up for the large losses in zinc which occur in the new-born baby, as a response to the stresses of birth.

ZINC AND VITAMIN A

Zinc is vital for maintaining proper levels of circulating vitamin A. This is because it is required in order to make a vitamin A carrier in the liver. Zinc deficiency has therefore been shown in animals to cause vitamin A deficiency, making it doubly important in pregnancy (5).

NUTRITION AND GROWTH IN CHILDREN

That zinc deficiency can cause stunted growth in children has been known since 1963, but just how much of a role zinc plays in short children is still uncertain. In a study designed to answer this vital question, 13 children between the ages of seven and 13, who had been found to have low zinc status in the hair, were given 50 or 100 mg of zinc a day. In those children whose hair zinc levels rose there was a significant increase in growth rate. Growth hormones produced by the body also increased with extra zinc (6). Zinc is needed in such large amounts by the growing foetus that it is not surprising to see a link between zinc status and growth (7). Supplementing zinc has been shown to increase growth rate, and is particularly pronounced in women who are heavy smokers. In one study, the average increase in birthweight of zinc-supplemented smoking mothers was 170 g or 6 oz (8). Zinc-deficient mothers have more complications at birth and the incidence of birth defects is higher. There also appears to be a connection between low zinc and increased risk for needing a Caesarean section (9,10).

WHEN SHOULD YOU START SUPPLEMENTATION?

When is zinc deficiency most dangerous and how late can you alleviate this potential problem? If animal studies can be related to us, the news is good. Zinc-deficient animals given zinc in the last quarter of pregnancy produce heavier young. Also, poor appetite, so often caused by zinc deficiency in infants, is corrected by late pregnancy zinc supplementation. Obviously it's better to start supplementing zinc even before conception, but it's never too late to start (11).

WHAT SORT OF ZINC IS BEST?

Zinc is highest in foods from animal sources, although it appears to be equally well absorbed from vegetable sources as well. In one study, zinc from animal or vegetable sources was given to see whether there was any change to zinc utilization. No distinction was found between animal and plant sources, with about 25 per cent of the available zinc in the diet being absorbed by pregnant women (12). Later studies have shown that zinc absorption does in fact go up substantially towards the end of pregnancy.

But it isn't just zinc which affects the birthweight of babies. Any form of malnutrition is likely to do the same thing. Poor nutrition during or before pregnancy may result in slower multiplication of cells, and therefore a slower rate of growth. Famines in Leningrad, Holland and Germany well illustrate the importance of nutrition. During the Leningrad famine in 1942 49 per cent of births were for babies weighing less than 5 lb 9 oz compared to the normal level in Britain of 6.9 per cent of births. Far more striking is the evidence from Holland during the Dutch hunger winter in 1944. Statistics show us that the incidence of perinatal mortality, stillbirths and underweight babies went up not so much for women who were pregnant during the famine, but for women who conceived during this period. The graph below illustrates this point clearly by showing how infant deaths during the first six days were substantially higher for those infants conceived during times of malnutrition.

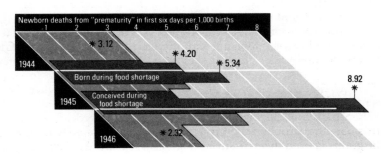

So, if you're thinking of getting pregnant, get 'zinced' first. A good daily intake from supplements is 20 mg. Zinc sulphate, zinc orotate, zinc gluconate or zinc amino-acid chelate are all well absorbed, but make sure you're taking 20 mg of the elemental level, not 20 mg of the compound. For example, zinc orotate 100 mg only provides 10 mg of zinc and 90 mg of orotate, so don't get caught out by this sleight of hand! Zinc absorption doubles when adequate levels of B6 are present in the diet. So it is often best to take zinc with vitamin B6.

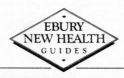

EBURY
NEW HEALTH
GUIDES

CHAPTER 6

PREVENTING PROBLEMS IN PREGNANCY

WHATEVER people tell you, there are a number of minor health problems that can and frequently do occur in pregnancy. By knowing what these are and taking simple precautionary measures you can often prevent these occurring, or at least alleviate the problems.

PREGNANCY SICKNESS

During the first three months of pregnancy all the organs of the baby are completely formed. It is during this period – and, of course, before conception – that optimum nutrition is most important. Yet many women experience continual sickness and don't feel like eating healthily.

Misnamed 'morning' sickness, this condition has been accepted as normal during the early part of pregnancy. The most common signs and symptoms associated with pregnancy sickness are nausea, usually worse on an empty stomach, and often triggered by smells of certain foods or perfumes; retching first thing in the morning or before meals; vomiting after eating; aversions to some foods and cravings for others; a metallic taste in the mouth; a feeling of hunger even when feeling nauseous; and relief from nausea by eating.

Pregnancy sickness is one example of a condition which usually only manifests in women whose nutritional status is less than optimum. Probably caused by an increase in a hormone called human chorionic gonadotrophin (HCG), women with poor diets are particularly at risk (1). This hormone is produced by the developing placenta from the moment of conception. It usually reaches its peak around nine to 10 weeks after the last period, and declines by week 14 to 16. Although it is produced later in pregnancy, the quantities present are far less. In very undernourished mothers HCG may not be produced in sufficient quantities at all, which may explain why women who miscarry early in pregnancy are less likely to experience any pregnancy sickness. On the other hand, very well-nourished women appear to ride the storm of these hormonal changes with little or no symptoms of nausea at all.

Other possible explanations for nausea or sickness involve the body trying to eliminate toxins, and also difficulty maintaining blood sugar balance. According to nutritionist Heather Bampfylde, toxins build up in your body during the night and the mechanism that helps to eliminate these needs B6 to work properly. Women low in vitamin B6 do have a greater risk of suffering from pregnancy sickness (2).

DIET TO PREVENT PREGNANCY SICKNESS

The best diet to prevent pregnancy sickness is explained more fully in Chapter 9 but the real keys to avoiding pregnancy sickness are:

- Always eat breakfast preferably containing some protein foods, like yoghurt or eggs.
- Eat small meals and frequent snacks of fruit and seeds. There is no limit to how much fresh fruit you can eat in a day.
- Avoid all sugar and refined foods.
- Avoid high-fat junk food, containing long lists of additives and preservatives.
- Decrease your intake of dried fruit or undiluted fruit juice, both of which provide concentrated sugar.
- Drink plenty of water between meals.
- Avoid or decrease your intake of coffee and tea.
- Avoid all alcohol and cigarettes.

NUTRIENTS TO PREVENT PREGNANCY SICKNESS

During pregnancy, the need for vitamin B6, B12, folic acid, iron and zinc all increase, and extra supplements of these usually stop even the worst cases of pregnancy sickness. Vitamin B6 is poorly supplied in the average diet. The RDA for B6 in America is 2 mg and most of us get less than this. However, during pregnancy minimal needs are at least 3 mg and often 100 mg is needed to stop pregnancy sickness. The same is true for vitamin B12. The RDA is 1 mcg, but 250 mcg of B12 is usually needed to prevent nausea in pregnancy. In the absence of any signs of deficiency other than pregnancy sickness I recommend my clients to take 100 mg of B6, 250 mcg of B12 and 400 mcg of folic acid. Normally, symptoms will disappear within two weeks, at which point these doses can be halved.

The mineral zinc may also be implicated in pregnant women who feel nauseous and go off food. According to Dr Pfeiffer and Nim Barnes of the Foresight organization for pre-conceptual care, 'The nauseated woman is usually deficient in both zinc and B6. Both are needed for growing tissues of any kind and the foetus and uterus make extra-ordinary demands on the mother's supply. Vitamin B6 has been used for nausea and vomiting in pregnancy with some success. We have had many pregnant patients who had difficulties with previous pregnancies go through a pregnancy on a zinc and B6 regime with no difficulties.' The minimum need for zinc during pregnancy is 20 mg a day while the average diet supplies less than 10 mg. So zinc supplementation is a must during pregnancy and doubly important if you experience nausea.

ANAEMIA

Mild anaemia may be present in one in three pregnant women. The symptoms include pallor, tiredness, a sore tongue and a feeling almost as if there's a weight on your shoulders. It is usually the result of a low level of iron in the blood protein haemoglobin, although B12, folic acid, manganese and B6 deficiency can also result in anaemia. Supplementing 20 mg of iron in the ferrous, not ferric, form (for example, ferrous sulphate) should alleviate this problem. Occasionally, 40 mg may be required. Your doctor should prescribe this for you. B12 deficiency anaemia is called pernicious anaemia. The symptoms of this can be masked by supplementing folic acid, so if folic acid is supplemented, B12 needs to be taken as well.

BACKACHE

If your posture is bad before pregnancy it's going to get worse during pregnancy and this can lead to backache. The tendons supporting the back become softer in pregnancy due to increased levels of the hormone progesterone. As the baby grows, your centre of gravity is pushed further forwards and, to compensate, many women push their shoulders back and their tummies out, putting strain on the back.

In pregnancy it is particularly important to maintain good posture. Imagine you are held up by a string attached to the top of your head, and keep your shoulders relaxed. When sitting don't slouch, and if you feel you need some support for the lower back, put a cushion between you and the back of the chair. Try to avoid lifting heavy objects. When you do lift don't do it by bending over and straining the back muscles.

Instead, bend your knees and keep your back straight, taking the weight with your thigh muscles.

CONSTIPATION

Many people imagine their abdominal organs – stomach, liver, pancreas, bladder and intestines – live in spacious surroundings. Actually, they are closely packed together. The arrival of a baby plus placenta, enlarged uterus and fluid, is a very tight fit and results in less room for the intestines, stomach and bladder to expand. For many women this means a greater chance of constipation since the faecal matter in the large intestine is more compressed and the muscles have less room to keep the contents moving along. The answer is not to take laxatives, but to make sure your diet is especially high in fluids and fibre and low in mucus-forming foods. Dairy produce, eggs and meat are especially mucus forming and tend to make faecal matter more compacted and harder to pass along. On the other hand, fruits, vegetables, grains, lentils and beans are high in fibre and this fibre absorbs fluid, making the resulting faecal matter light and bulky and easier to pass. It is a good idea to drink about a pint of water a day, either as it is or in diluted fruit juice. While it isn't strictly needed to maintain the water balance of the body it does help relieve constipation. By the way, drinking more water will in no way encourage fluid retention.

HEARTBURN

It is usual in the last months of pregnancy to experience some heartburn. This is due to pressure of the enlarged uterus on the stomach. There is no magical cure, other than to avoid the foods that cause you heartburn, and to eat small amounts more often rather than having big meals. Many women find it necessary to sleep slightly propped up towards the end of pregnancy.

ECLAMPSIA AND PRE-ECLAMPSIA

Eclampsia is a disease that only occurs in pregnancy. The first early warning sign of pre-eclampsia is raised blood pressure. The blood pressure may be only slightly raised to 140/90. This may be accompanied by slight oedema (swelling) in the ankles and protein in the urine; it occurs in 5 per cent of pregnancies. Once the pregnancy is over the symptoms all go away. However, eclampsia can be very serious indeed, causing fits which can endanger the life of the mother and baby. It is for this reason that regular check-ups are very important since women with pre-eclampsia don't necessarily feel ill.

The condition is thought to be connected with incomplete formation of the placenta. The placenta keeps mother and baby's blood supply separate, preventing the mother's immune system reacting to the foetus as a foreign body as it would to a virus or cancer cell. This mechanism may be at fault due to a malformed placenta. The larger the baby becomes the less well this poorly functioning system can manage, which is why pre-eclampsia occurs towards the end of a pregnancy. Mothers who have had pre-eclampsia in the first child are usually much better in the second. This is thought to be due to an adaptation of the immune system. According to medical researchers Ylastalo and Ylikorkala, an exaggerated rise in copper may also be a factor in pre-eclamptic toxaemia (1).

HIGH BLOOD PRESSURE

This is unlikely to occur in those who have had no previous history of high blood pressure. If the blood pressure rises above 160/100 the person must be carefully monitored. This usually accompanies oedema (fluid retention) in face, hands, ankles and abdomen. There is no known medical cure, although bed rest often helps. Drugs are avoided where possible since these can affect supply of blood to baby.

LEG CRAMPS

Cramps are almost invariably caused by an imbalance of calcium and magnesium. These minerals, as well as sodium and potassium, are called electrolytes because they control the electrical balance that turns muscle cells on and off. Cramps are caused by muscles going into contraction. Deficiency of calcium, magnesium or sodium can cause this; however, sodium deficiency is extremely rare. Because of the baby's demand for calcium and magnesium to make healthy bones, pregnant women often become deficient. While milk products are particularly high in calcium they are almost completely devoid of magnesium. Green leafy vegetables, nuts and seeds are quite good sources of both calcium and magnesium. However, eating more of these foods often doesn't provide enough calcium and magnesium to banish cramps completely. A dietary supplement of dolomite, which is calcium and magnesium, is therefore advisable.

STRETCH MARKS

The skin on the abdomen does a remarkable stretching job in pregnancy. If the skin loses its natural elasticity stretch marks may develop.
Stretch marks on the stomach, thighs, breasts, hips or shoulder girdle
are one of the signs of zinc deficiency so adequate zinc intake is crucial.
Vitamin C is needed to make collagen, the intercellular glue, and
vitamin E helps to keep skin supple. Applying vitamin E oil or cream is
helpful during the last weeks of pregnancy and after the birth to
encourage the skin to contract. Most of all, abdominal muscles must be
kept strong throughout pregnancy and afterwards otherwise you will
be left with a flabby tummy. It takes many months to return abdominal
muscles to their former strength so persevere with the abdominal
exercises.

VARICOSE VEINS

The development of varicose veins during pregnancy is not at all
uncommon. This is caused by the restricted flow of blood returning
from the feet and legs in the groin area due to the baby and is also due to
constipation. All the blood vessels in the legs lead to one big vein in the
groin. If this is compressed the blood must return along different
routes. This can cause small veins on the surface of the legs to become
enlarged. The result is prominent veins that may become varicose
veins.

The secret of avoiding these unsightly blood vessels is to keep the
veins in good shape and to minimize the restriction of blood flow.
Vitamin C is needed to make collagen which keeps the arteries supple.
Vitamin B3 helps to dilate the blood vessels, while vitamin E and the
essential fatty acid EPA (high in fish) thin the blood and help to
transport oxygen in the blood. A high-fibre diet helps to reduce
constipation, removing additional pressure on the main vein in the
groin area, and regular exercise helps to stimulate proper circulation.

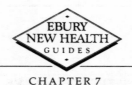

CHAPTER 7

PREVENTING ALLERGIES IN YOUR CHILD

Virtually no baby survives the first six months without an allergic reaction. This may manifest as an unexplained rash, colic or cold-like symptoms. But whether this is a rare or common event depends very much on the mother's diet during pregnancy and breast feeding, as well as the kind of foods the baby is weaned on to.

WHAT IS AN ALLERGY?

In the loosest sense of the word an allergy is any unusual reaction to a food, chemical or inhalant such as pollen. Most of these reactions are immunological, which means that the substance, called an allergen, causes the immune system to mount an allergic attack to eliminate this 'alien'. In immunology jargon the offending food is called an 'antigen' and the immune cells produce 'antibodies' to get rid of it.

Food allergens are most commonly protein, which theoretically should never get through the intestinal wall. The processes of digestion should break them down into amino acids, which are the building blocks of protein, to which the immune system won't respond. However, new-born babies are far more likely to react allergically, especially during the first three months of life. This is because their intestinal wall is not yet fully developed and is therefore more permeable to large food particles passing through and causing a reaction. There is some evidence that atopic children, which means those with a slight eczema, asthma or allergic rhinitis (a tendency which runs in families), have more permeable gut walls and therefore are hypersensitive (1). However, all children, especially babies, have increased allergic sensitivity. In one study in which 10 children aged five years were given the food additive tartrazine (E 102), used to colour drinks and foods yellow/orange, all developed itching within two to eight hours (2).

The foods that most often cause a reaction are the foods eaten most frequently. The top allergy-provoking foods are milk, eggs, yeast, oranges, sugar, food colourings, all other grains, chocolate and nuts.

ALLERGIES START IN THE WOMB

According to some new research allergies may even start in the womb. Babies who are uncomfortably active in the womb may be trying to tell you they don't like the room service! This may be the very first sign of hyperactivity and food allergy. So the place to start preventing food allergies in children is with the mother's diet during and, if possible, before pregnancy.

PREVENTING ALLERGIES IN YOUR CHILD

In order to minimize the risk of your child developing allergies the first step is to identify your own food allergies, if any, and eliminate those substances that cause a pronounced reaction and 'rotate' those foods which cause a minor reaction. A rotation (see page 47) diet means that you eat the food less frequently and certainly not every day. Most rotation diets are based on eating the food every fifth day and allergists believe that this practice actually desensitizes the individual from that food. But how do you find out what you are allergic to?

DISCOVERING YOUR ALLERGIES

Discovering your allergies is like detective work. You can work out your potential suspects by asking yourself four questions.

1 What foods (or drinks) do I suspect that I react badly to?
2 What foods do I eat at least once if not more every day?
3 What foods would I find hardest to give up?
4 Which of these foods are in the top allergens?

A food that fulfils all these criteria is a strong suspect. To test whether you do react to these foods a simple pulse test can be done after avoiding the food for 15 days.

THE PULSE TEST FOR ALLERGIES

Avoid all the substances you suspect strictly for 28 days. And do check the contents of the foods you eat carefully to see whether they contain any of these ingredients. It is best to prepare yourself well by stocking up with your allergen-free foods before starting. Then do this simple pulse test:

1 Take your pulse at rest (after five minutes sitting down), for 60 seconds. Your pulse can be found inside the bony protuberance on the thumb side of your wrist (see illustration).
2 Then eat more than usual of the No 1 food.
3 Take your pulse after 10, 30 and 60 minutes. Make sure you take your pulse at rest for the duration of 60 seconds.
4 Keep a record of any symptoms over the next 24 hours.

If your pulse increases by 10 points or if you have any noticeable symptoms within 24 hours, avoid this substance and wait 48 hours before testing the next item on your list.

If your pulse does not increase by 10 points and you have no change in symptoms, reintroduce this food (in moderation) into your diet, and proceed with the same test for the next food.

AVOIDING YOUR ALLERGENS

If you get a clear increase in pulse rate, or symptoms of a reaction, these substances are best avoided completely. This is little problem if you simply find you react to chocolate or coffee. But it can be quite awkward if you react to more staple foods like wheat or milk produce.

If you suspect wheat, stay off all wheat-containing items like bread, cakes, biscuits, pasta, sauces and cereals. Alternatives are oat cakes, rice cakes, rye crispbread, sauces made with corn flour, corn- or oat-based cereals and pastry made with corn and almond meal instead of wheat.

While some people react to all grains, others just react to wheat. This may be due to the gluten content, which is the prime protein in wheat. Bread often causes the strongest reaction which may be because the gluten content is high and the process of kneading the bread activates the gluten. There is some suggestion that modern hybrids of wheat have changed the protein structure, and it is this 'new' wheat that we react to. (Dr Nadia Coates at Springhill Farm has been recultivating the wheat they grow to end up with grain similar to that used by our ancestors and has found that patients react less allergically to their products. Springhill bread is widely available in health food shops.)

If you are avoiding milk stay off all milk, cheese, yoghurt, butter, chocolate and foods containing milk produce. Good alternatives are soya milk, or nut cream, made by blending nuts with water (cashews are particularly good). Drink herb teas that do not require milk, and have more free-range eggs if cheese is a major source for your protein.

Since your calcium intake is important during pregnancy you are advised to supplement calcium as well as eating a diet rich in green leafy vegetables, seeds and almonds. The best level of calcium supplementation is explained in the next chapter. Provided these indications are followed, there is no danger in avoiding milk products.

Many people are unable to digest milk sugar (lactose) because they lack the enzyme lactase. However, lactase deficiency itself is not the likely reason for milk allergy. Many people are lactase deficient, particularly people of African and Indian origin. According to Dr Passmore from Edinburgh this doesn't prevent the enjoyment of milk. 'There is of course a substantial minority who cannot tolerate even small amounts of milk. To identify the underlying causes of their intolerance is a challenge for future research, but it is not due to intestinal lactase.' (3) These few react to particular proteins in milk. The more the nature of the milk has been changed, the less likely they are to react. Butter, being primarily fat, is often tolerated by the milk allergic. Carnation milk, yoghurt and cheese may also be tolerated in small amounts. Some people don't react so strongly to goat's milk as cow's milk, and again this is probably due to different proteins in the milk.

ROTATION DIETS

On a food rotation diet, the offending food is eaten only every fifth day and this appears to build up a tolerance to the food. For example, if you react to milk, wheat and oranges, then this would be a rotation diet for you.

Monday	Tuesday	Wednesday	Thursday	Friday	Saturday	Sunday
Wheat	*Milk*	*Oranges*		*Wheat*	*Milk*	*Oranges*

On those days specified you could eat as much wheat, milk or oranges as you care to; on the middle day all possible allergens would be avoided.

BREAST FEEDING PROTECTS AGAINST ALLERGY

The breast-fed baby has some protection against allergies because the mother passes on antibodies and immune cells in her milk. These act like intestinal paint, preventing the potential allergens from crossing the intestinal barrier. However, a breast-fed baby can still react to foods consumed by the mother so the protection isn't complete.

ALLERGIES IN CHILDREN

Is your baby, or will he be, subject to colic, wind, sleeplessness, irritability, eczema and later asthma, runny nose, coughing, muscle aches, bed wetting, oedema, persistent infections, hyperactivity, hives, rashes? Well, hopefully not, but these are all symptoms of allergy which every mother would do well to be aware of. Many babies react to a food or material that suits a brother or sister. Often these symptoms occur singly, then stop and a different symptom appears.

A mother's food addictions can be passed on before birth and bottle feeding allows foreign cow proteins into an unprotected neonatal gut.

Weaning is the next stage at which food allergies can be acquired. Well-known babycare books state that a baby can be given his first new foods at any age between one and six months, but research shows that the incidence of allergy increases by weaning early.

Eggs and cereals are almost invariably the first foods to be given and yet these, along with milk, are the most common offenders for causing allergy in infants. For some infants, giving these foods, or the way that you give them, can be wrong. Eggs are advised and are sometimes given after one month because they are rich in iron. This is usually unnecessary as the baby's iron supply should be good for six months. The iron is in the yolk and it is only the yolk that should be given from six to 12 months (the white contains the foreign proteins that could cause allergy in a sensitive gut).

Rice is the least allergenic cereal, followed by oats and barley, so if you must give cereal first, rice is the one to start with; however, variety is the main way to avoid allergies and, for this reason, after allowing a baby to get used to a new food it is best to rotate the cereals, e.g. rice on day 1, oats on day 2, wheat on day 3 and corn or barley on day 4.

IMMUNE POWER

Avoiding allergens is only half of the story. The other half involves boosting your immune power to reduce allergic potential in the first place.

Our body's defence against alien invaders, including food proteins, is called the immune system. It consists of various cells called anti-bodies, macrophages and lymphocytes with a search and destroy mission against defective cells, viruses or food particles that find their way uninvited inside us. For example, when we are exposed to a food protein that we've seen before, the B-Lymphocytes release specific 'antibodies' designed to attach only to the offending 'antigen', in this case an allergen which triggers the allergy. Meanwhile, macrophages and T-Lymphocytes are beckoned to the scene of the crime. These engulf the invader and begin to ingest and destroy it by releasing all sorts of chemicals. More than 50 chemicals secreted from macrophages have been identified so far. They also produce 'free radicals', dangerous forms of oxygen which destroy the invader, but must themselves be destroyed once their job is over. This is done with anti-oxidants, like vitamin C and E, and anti-oxidant enzymes, like glutathione peroxidase, which is dependent on selenium. As well as lymphocytes that boost the immune response there are ones that stop the reaction and restore peace once the invasion is over. These are called suppressor T-Lymphocytes.

And if that wasn't enough already, there are additional components called NK (Natural Killer) lymphocytes, and interferon, which all play a part in winning the battles that go on every day inside us. NK cells are our strongest ally against cancer cells. Interferon also suppresses cancer cell growth.

THE MICRONUTRIENT IMMUNE BOOSTERS

A weak immune system can result in frequent colds and infections. But more dangerous than this is an over-aggressive immune system that doesn't know when to stop reacting and what to react to. Food allergy is an example of the immune system over-reacting.

A strong immune system means a greater resistance both to infections and colds, but also to allergies. And there is no stronger way to fortify your immune system than through optimum nutrition.

The components of our white army are made primarily of protein and adequate protein nutrition is vital for a strong immune system. Protein deficiency has been shown to reduce lymphocyte and interferon production and to prevent the destruction of cancer cells. Since fat and cholesterol both weaken the immune system it is best to derive protein from lean meat or a vegetarian source.

B vitamin deficiency has long been known to affect immunity. People suffering from pantothenic acid or B6 deficiency have atrophy of the thymus gland and spleen, which is where the basic material for lymphocytes and macrophages is made. Severe B6 deficiency results in no antibody formation at all! Ideal intake for B6 goes up with protein intake and doses well in excess of 100 mg are often required for maximum immune power. The same is also true for pantothenic acid (B5), where up to 2,000 mg have been used. These B vitamins should always be taken with a B complex and mineral formula providing zinc and manganese.

Both folic acid and vitamin B12 are needed for proper production of lymphocytes, the white blood cells, as well as being vital for red blood cell health and the transport of oxygen. But most important of all the vitamins is vitamin C. Despite some damning research of vitamin C's anti-cold properties, there is no doubt that vitamin C plays a key role in immunity. Animals deficient in vitamin C produce less T-Lymphocytes and, when vitamin C is supplemented, produce more. These white blood cells travel faster to the scene of the crime when vitamin C is present.

C AND E WORK TOGETHER

Vitamin C's potency depends in part on the amount of vitamin E available. Also an anti-oxidant, vitamin E appears to be freed from its complex with the dangerous oxide radicals to fight another battle when high levels of vitamin C are also present. Vitamin E in turn protects vitamin A from oxidation. But most of all, large doses (800 to 1,600 ius per day) have been shown to improve immune response, increasing B and T-Lymphocytes. In animals exposed to infection, vitamin E gives a four-fold increase in survival rate. The most active form of vitamin E is d-alpha tocopherol (not dl-alpha tocopherol) which is a natural source. Other tocopherols exist which may also have a role to play. Nuts and seeds provide mixed tocopherols. Make sure these are fresh to minimize the amount of rancid oils present.

STRENGTHENING YOUR INSIDE SKIN

Before allergens can do damage, they must cross the first line of defence – your inside skin. This may be the lungs or the intestinal tract. Either way, vitamin A strengthens these membranes against invaders. It also boosts production of virus-digesting enzymes and, when given in doses of 30,000 to 50,000 ius to surgery patients, prevents the post-operative drop in lymphocyte counts which leaves the patient open to infection.

But vitamin A itself can be toxic – at least in the animal form called retinol. Beta-carotene, the vegetable form found in orange-coloured foods including carrots, beetroot, apricots, peaches, and green leafy vegetables, is quite safe in large doses. However, beta-carotene is half as potent as retinol and, as the dose increases, less is converted to the active form by the liver. This mechanism is probably nature's way of preventing toxicity in animals eating large quantities of vitamin A rich fruits and vegetables.

THE ZINC-COLD CONNECTION

It is clear that zinc has a profound influence on immune responses, reports one of Britain's leading experts on nutrition and immunity, Dr Stephen Davies. 'When zinc is deficient, children become prone to infections.' The thymus also atrophies, according to work by Dr Golden in Jamaica. So pronounced is this effect, that after only 10 days of zinc supplementation at a level of 2 mg per kg bodyweight, thymus size measurably increases. Another study reported a 221 per cent increase in T-Lymphocyte function once zinc deficiency had been corrected.

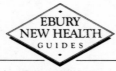

CHAPTER 8

GETTING FIT NOT FAT

THE last thing you want to do in pregnancy is put your feet up and start eating more. Keeping fit in pregnancy will help your labour tremendously and keeping trim will also increase your chances of a healthy baby. But it's a lot easier if you start your pregnancy fit and not fat, rather than trying to get it together once you realize you are pregnant. First, let's look at exercise.

KEEPING FIT IN PREGNANCY

If you are already doing exercise on a regular basis there is no reason for you to stop when you're pregnant. Whether it's running, swimming, aerobics or dance classes, keep it up. These exercises are all excellent 'aerobic' exercises if done properly, which means they demand your body to take in and use oxygen more efficiently. This improves the health of your heart and arteries, which is all good news for your baby. Giving birth has been likened, in terms of sheer physical exertion, to running a marathon. Of course, the longer the labour the harder you work. So it pays to be aerobically fit.

If you are generally unfit, pregnancy is not the time to leap with gay abandon into strenuous heart-pounding exercise. However, it is the time to gradually increase your level of exercise. This can first be done by going for brisk walks, preferably involving the odd hill. Going swimming or attending beginners' aerobics classes, leaving out the hard bits, is the next thing to do. Exercise should be fun so choose something you enjoy.

STRENGTHENING YOUR STOMACH MUSCLES

All these stamina-building exercises have the added advantage of developing your abdominal muscles. This is absolutely crucial for the birth, but even more so for afterwards for a speedy recovery. During pregnancy the abdominal muscles get severely stretched and unless you do some form of exercise to maintain abdominal muscle tone you are very likely to suffer from backache, have a harder time in labour, and end up with a bigger belly after the event.

If your current exercise programme doesn't include abdominal exercises it is worth setting aside five minutes of every day to strengthen these muscles. Here's what to do: Lie on your back on the floor with your knees bent. Tuck your hips under, pressing your back down against the floor, repeat as often and frequently as possible. When you feel comfortable and confident doing this combine the tuck with a small lift of your upper body, bringing your hands to touch your knees. First touch both right and left hand on the corresponding knee, then touch your left hand on your right knee and vice versa.

PELVIC FLOOR EXERCISES

Another exercise to do each day is the pelvic floor exercise. To discover where your pelvic floor muscles are, stop the flow of urine when you are passing water – you will feel the muscles contracting and relaxing. If you stop and start the flow continually, you will be exercising your pelvic floor. This action of continually clenching and releasing your pelvic floor can be done completely discreetly while sitting at a desk or even waiting for a bus – it is important to do it as frequently as possible.

WHEN TO STOP EXERCISING

You can go on exercising in pregnancy until your body tells you to stop. The fitter you are, the later this will be. In fact many people exercise right up to the end of pregnancy. Usually it is not the physical inability that stops people exercising, but feeling tired.

I have some words of caution, however. Firstly, there is no doubt that big bumps or falls or any physical trauma can cause a miscarriage. This is more likely to occur earlier in pregnancy so it is not a good idea to go skiing for the first time in the first three months or take up hang-gliding while you're pregnant! Secondly, the risk of injury to joints is also greater in pregnancy, for two reasons. The extra pounds of weight you are carrying put more of a strain on the weight-bearing joints (your hips, knees and ankles) as well as your back. Also, the hormonal changes in pregnancy loosen ligaments and this helps to free up the pelvis which is vital for delivering the baby so one side effect of this is that you are more likely to dislocate a joint during pregnancy.

EXERCISE HELPS YOU TO LOSE WEIGHT

As long as you bear these cautions in mind together with a modicum of common sense, pregnancy is a great time to keep fit. In fact it is also an excellent time to get less fat. Although you should gain weight during pregnancy, by doing the right exercise and eating the right diet many people find that after the birth they are slimmer than before.

A study at the University of Vermont in Canada examined the effects of exercise on weight during pregnancy in a group of 228 women. The women were divided into three groups: those who did aerobic exercise (aerobics, running or cross-country skiing) at least three times a week for 30 minutes; those who exercised six times a week or more for an hour or more; and those who did minimal exercise. 60 per cent of women in the 'maximum' exercise group and 68 per cent of those in the 'minimal' exercise group had stopped exercising by the twentieth week. The reasons given were fatigue, lack of time, lower abdominal discomfort, musculoskeletal injury, nausea and general concern. Even so, these women gained on average 10 lb less during pregnancy.

HOW MUCH WEIGHT SHOULD YOU GAIN?

It is normal to gain 8 lb in weight by the end of the first 20 weeks, and to gain about a pound per week after that. That makes a total weight gain of around 28 lb or 2 st. But not all this is you! In fact, your weight gain shouldn't be more than 8 lb of fat which is there as a reserve to help ensure your and the baby's energy supply is adequate. The rest is made up of the baby, the placenta, increased size of breasts and uterus, increased blood volume and extra body fluids. The chart below shows you how these increase during pregnancy.

WEIGHT GAIN DURING PREGNANCY
(Hytten & Leitch 1971)

	10 weeks	20 weeks	30 weeks	40 weeks
Total weight gain	1.4 lb	8.8 lb	18.7 lb	27.5 lb
Foetus and placenta	0.12	1.6	5.6	10
Uterus and breasts	0.37	1.7	2.6	2.9
Blood	0.22	1.3	2.9	2.6
Extracellular fluid	–	–	–	2.6
Fat	0.71	4.2	7.7	8.8

These are only the average gains in weight and people vary enormously. If your weight gain is more, check you are not overeating or possibly suffering from oedema, caused by water retention. If your weight gain is less than half this amount it is important to check that you are eating enough. Since the more important measure is whether the baby is growing, measuring your waist is a better indication than your weight.

HOW MUCH EXTRA DO YOU NEED TO EAT?

Most diets for pregnant women are based on their needing an extra 300 calories a day – a 10 per cent increase in calorie intake. But recent research has calculated that all the extra calories a woman needs is 50 a day (2). This is less than an extra apple a day, so you don't have to 'eat for two'. It isn't how much you eat but what you eat that is most important.

In fact, one study showed that fat women had smaller babies than women of the right weight (3). Conversely, two studies have shown that mothers of equivalent weight, but less well nourished, have smaller babies. So provided your diet is good and you take the right vitamin and mineral supplements there is no need to eat substantially more during pregnancy. Your body should tell you what you need.

KEEPING ACTIVE

The best way to prevent extra pounds creeping on is to keep active. This will keep up your metabolic rate and help you to burn off unwanted fat. Don't sit at home for nine months. It's a recipe for eating too much. Continue working or get a part-time job. Alternatively, turn your garden into the garden of Eden or decorate your house from top to bottom. Do the things that you won't be able to do with a young baby around. It may be your last chance for a holiday abroad for a while, so get a good holiday. On the nutrition programme explained in this book you'll have plenty of energy to use up so make the most of it.

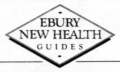

CHAPTER 9

THE BETTER PREGNANCY DIET

Even if your diet is perfectly adequate when you're not pregnant there's no reason to assume it is adequate when you are. At any time of stress, which includes puberty, menopause, menstruation, but most of all pregnancy, nutritional needs are greatest. These needs will be drawn on and if you don't have enough nutrients in the bank you'll go overdrawn. By having a better pregnancy diet your nutrient intake, although perhaps higher than your everyday need, will be sufficiently high to meet these times of extra need.

Consider the experiences of Mary. She came to me with symptoms of headaches, digestive problems, excessive sleeping and most of all exhaustion. Her continual tiredness often made her feel depressed. She'd done the rounds of various doctors who had run this and that blood test and found nothing wrong. Her diet was by all accounts much better than average, but here she was suffering from all the signs of multiple vitamin and mineral deficiency. What was causing this?

The answer was simple. Over the past 10 years she had produced and breast-fed six babies. That means that in the past eight years she had been feeding two people! Her diet just wasn't giving her enough nutrients. With a few dietary changes and vitamin supplements all her symptoms improved within four weeks.

THE PROTEIN MYTH

During pregnancy protein is used more efficiently. Most of our protein is used to make the cells that we're made of. The excess gets converted into energy. In pregnancy, less protein is used for energy and more is stored for use by the baby. For this reason urea levels in the blood, which are an indication of protein breakdown, often drop in pregnancy. This protein storing means that the need for increased protein is spread over the entire pregnancy.

The recommended intake for protein goes up 11 per cent in pregnancy. On top of the normal protein requirement of 54 g we need an extra 6 g a day maximum. Some nutritionists consider that this estimate is too high. The overall need for protein depends on both the quality of the protein and the dietary intake of vitamins and minerals which determines how well you use protein. So if you eat good quality protein and are not vitamin or mineral deficient you can afford to eat less than this. The absolute minimum requirement for protein during pregnancy is 49 g a day. A list of the foods that contain good quality protein is on page 113. The common belief that animal produce is the only source of protein is wrong. By combining vegetarian sources of protein you can get excellent quality protein, without the disadvantage of a high fat intake which is associated with eating too much red meat.

THE GOOD AND THE BAD FATS

It may surprise you to hear that fat can be good or bad. In the last decade more and more has been discovered about the role of certain essential fats that appear to have a hormone-like control on many body mechanisms including sex hormones, allergic reactions and health of the arteries. These essential fats are linoleic and linolenic acid. They are highest in sunflower, sesame, safflower, soya and maize oil. We need one to two tablespoons a day, and you can get a substantial amount if you eat seeds and nuts. There is one problem, however. Both these fats are part of a family of unsaturated fats. This means that they are particularly prone to damage from oxidation, which we know of as rancidity. Any heating process causes oxidation so these oils need to be extracted without heat. So make sure you get cold-pressed sunflower, sesame or safflower oil. Also, don't cook with them. They should be used only for salad dressings, mayonnaises, spreads and any other non-heated use. Keep them in the fridge, as this helps to prevent rancidity.

Linoleic and linolenic acid present in these oils go through various stages of transformation inside us before they can be of use. Linoleic acid turns into Gamma Linolenic Acid or GLA. GLA is found in a number of plants like the evening primrose, blackcurrant seeds and in the herb borage. Extracts from these plants are sold as dietary supplements. Linolenic acid eventually turns into Eicosapentaenoic Acid or EPA for short. This is found in oily fish like mackerel and is also high in cod liver oil. Both GLA and EPA eventually turn into hormone-like substances called prostaglandins. It is these that help balance sex hormones among other things, and their therapeutic use has been successful for PMT, eczema and other skin conditions, heart disease and migraine. Essential fats are also found in most cells of the body, especially those in the brain. They are also used to insulate nerves. (Multiple sclerosis is a condition where this insulation breaks down resulting in loss of muscle control.) So make sure you get some essential fats in your diet.

Saturated fats, which come mainly from animal sources, differ from unsaturated fats in that they tend to be solid at room temperature, can't make prostaglandins, and are less likely to become rancid. They are ideal padding and insulating material and can be used for energy, but most of us eat far too much. And there are no exceptions for pregnancy. A low-saturated-fat diet is a healthy diet, so that means less meat, butter, eggs, cheese, milk and high-fat convenience foods. Just by eating lean meat, low-fat cheese and skimmed milk you can help reduce your fat intake. Frying an onion increases its fat content 32 times. So avoid frying as much as possible and grill or bake instead. Ironically, if you do fry it is probably better to use a very small amount of butter or olive oil (which is closer to being a saturated fat) than vegetable oil, since these fats are not easily oxidized and foods high in oxides are not good for you.

So which is better – butter or margarine? In truth, both should be avoided as much as possible. To make vegetable oils solid at room temperature these oils go through a process called hydrogenation. This changes the form of the oil and renders it unable to make prostaglandins. However, most margarines add back some unprocessed cold-pressed vegetable oils. The best margarines from this point of view are Vitaquell and Granose, both of which are widely available in health food shops.

NO SUGAR, THANKS

Probably the most important dietary change in pregnancy is to cut down on sugar. Not only is sugar bad for you and your baby but also most sources of sugar are 'empty calories' – they supply the calories but no nutrients to go with them. As much as two-thirds of most people's calorie intake is from empty-calorie foods consisting of refined grains, sugar and fat.

Very high levels of sugar in the form of glucose interfere with normal sugar metabolism, and can cause birth defects. The same effects do not appear with fructose or galactose which are the forms of sugar found in fruit and dairy produce (1). So if you have an uncontrollable sweet tooth, eat lots of fruit instead.

During pregnancy, many women become mildly hypoglycaemic. This means their blood sugar level fluctuates abnormally. They learn that eating sugary foods, or having another coffee (which causes the mobilization of sugar from the liver) makes them feel temporarily better. But 'temporarily' is the key word. Any regular overconsumption of sugar, alcohol, strong tea or coffee can lead to ever-worsening signs of hypoglycaemia. The symptoms include irritability, depression, dizziness, forgetfulness, fatigue, thirst and lack of sex drive. Does this sound like anybody you know?

The answer is to eat small, frequent meals containing either some protein or complex carbohydrate. Snack on sunflower seeds, oat cakes, pieces of fruit, rather than biscuits, sweets and cakes. If you suspect you may be hypoglycaemic, it is also a good idea to eat breakfast. This helps to raise the blood sugar level. Dilute fruit juices as these are fairly concentrated sweetness and watch out for transferring your sweet tooth into eating loads of dried fruit or honey under the guise that you've stopped eating sugar.

FIBRE

One of the difficulties most often encountered during pregnancy is constipation. Later on in pregnancy the baby will press on your abdomen, making it harder to eat a lot and making you prone to constipation. In pregnancy, a high-fibre diet is doubly important. High fibre diets soak up water in the intestines making faecal matter soft and bulky. This is easy for the muscles of the large intestine to move along. If your diet is high in sticky, mucusy foods like meat and milk and low in fibre, stools become more and more compact and harder to pass. In fact the word constipation comes from the Latin word *constipare*, meaning to pack together. High fibre doesn't mean just adding bran to a fibre-poor diet. It is far better to get your fibre from the foods you eat. All vegetables, grains, nuts, lentils and beans contain significant amounts of fibre. Don't have white rice or bread, have brown. Also, drink lots of water. You will find that you pass water more frequently in pregnancy because the baby also squashes your bladder.

Three typical days' menus for the Better Pregnancy Diet are given on pages 60 and 61.

DAY 1

BANANA BREAKFAST
A delicious combination of natural yoghurt, banana, wheatgerm, crunchy coconut and dates.

RAINBOW ROOT SALAD
A colourful combination of raw grated carrots, beetroots and parsnip with an island dressing made from tomatoes, tofu, mayonnaise, carrot and ground almonds.

SPAGHETTI NAPOLITANA
Wholemeal spaghetti with a sauce of carrots, tomatoes and mushrooms, flavoured with thyme. Serve with a generous sprinkling of Parmesan cheese and watercress salad.

RASPBERRY SORBET
Frozen raspberries and bananas liquidized to a smooth purée.

As snacks throughout the day – three pieces of fruit in season, including an apple eaten with a large chunk of Cheddar cheese. Drink Barleycup, dandelion coffee, Red Zinger, Lemon Mist or any of the other 'Celestial Seasonings' herb teas.

DAY 2

FRUIT MILKSHAKE
A delicious creamy purée of fruit (try peaches, strawberries, banana, fresh dates or even mango), ground almonds, vanilla essence and desiccated coconut, skimmed milk and ice.

BOILED EGG
Served with wholemeal toast.

LENTIL SOUP
A thick, nourishing combination of lentils and onions seasoned with vegetable stock. Served with coleslaw – chopped white cabbage and carrot with a mayonnaise and yoghurt dressing.

COURGETTE QUICKIE
Courgettes, tomatoes, onions and garlic with a crispy cheese and breadcrumb topping, served on a bed of brown rice with watercress or green salad.

APRICOT WHISK
A purée of apricots with low-fat curd cheese lightened with whisked egg whites.

As snacks throughout the day – plenty of fresh fruit in season. Drinks – as for day one or try some new herb teas – lemon verbena, peppermint or rosehip.

DAY 3

MUESLI WITH FRESH APPLE
Sugar-free muesli with chopped apple and milk.

FILLED BAKED POTATO
Baked potato stuffed with cottage cheese, chives and cucumber.

MUSHROOM PILAFF
Brown rice cooked with mushrooms, raisins and peas, flavoured with parsley and ginger. Serve with a tomato and beansprout salad followed by baked apple filled with dates.

As snacks throughout the day—three pieces of fresh fruit, a few nibbles of Cheddar cheese or almonds. Drink herb tea or coffee substitutes, like Bambu or instant chicory coffee.

How many vitamins and minerals does this sort of diet really provide? In the table on page 62 we've listed all the vitamins and minerals, together with fat, protein and carbohydrate content provided in the above daily menus. You'll see five columns: the Nutrients, the Recommended Daily Allowance, the Optimum Level, what the Average Diet provides and what the Optimum Diet above would provide. These need a little explaining.

1 The standard British Recommended Daily Allowances (RDAs) are used.
2 OLs (Optimum Levels) are those used at the Institute for Optimum Nutrition, based on current research and clinical findings.
3 The average diet is based on the Ministry of Agriculture's yearly National Food Survey, taking into account cooking losses.
4 This is the average intake from the three days' menus shown on the previous pages.

OPTIMUM NUTRITION VS BASIC NUTRITION

For every nutrient, government departments set a Recommended Daily Allowance (RDA). This is the figure you see on your cornflakes packet. The RDA is designed to prevent people getting obvious vitamin deficiency signs. However, these doses may not be optimum, they are just the basic requirements to prevent severe malnutrition. Optimum Levels vary from person to person, but I have set these at the levels that have been shown to maximize health. This means that at these levels enzymes dependent on these vitamins function optimally, that no small signs of deficiency occur, and the chances of a healthy pregnancy are maximized.

Nutrient	RDA[1]	OL[2]	Av.Diet[3]	Opt.Diet[4]
Total Calories	2,400	2,400	2,210	2,500
Protein	60 g	90 g	72 g	100 g
Carbohydrate	–	330 g	264 g	539 g
Fat	–	80 g	104 g	87 g
Saturated	–	26 g	46 g	29 g
Monounsaturated	–	>50 g	39 g	34 g
Polyunsaturated	–	<8 g	11 g	8 g
Fibre	–	35 g	20 g	39 g
Vitamins				
A	2,250 iu	7,500 iu	4,020 iu	41,000 iu
D	–	400 iu	2.99 mcg	213 iu
E	–	400 iu	?	24 iu
C	60 mg	2,000 mg	59 mg	250 mg
B1 (thiamine)	1 mg	25 mg	1.15 mg	2.5 mg
B2 (riboflavin)	1.6 mg	25 mg	1.87 mg	3.5 mg
B3 (niacin)	18 mg	50 mg	13.9 mg	27 mg
B5 (pantothenic acid)	–	50 mg	?	35 mg
B6 (pyridoxine)	–	100 mg	1.36 mg	21 mg
B12	–	50 mcg	6.6 mcg	16 mcg
Folic Acid	–	800 mcg	190 mcg	613 mcg
Biotin	–	200 mcg	*	*
Minerals				
Sodium	–	3,000 mg	12,000 mg	1,985 mg
Potassium	–	5,000 mg	4,000 mg	8,000 mg
Calcium	1,200 mg	1,200 mg	855 mg	1,600 mg
Magnesium	450 mg	600 mg	249 mg	677 mg
Iron	18 mg	18 mg	10.9 mg	27 mg
Zinc	–	20 mg	9.1 mg	13 mg
Chromium	–	50 mcg	20 mcg	*
Manganese	–	5 mg	3 mg	*
Selenium	–	25 mcg	*	*

*no available information.

This is well illustrated by the experiment which shows what happens to animals given different doses of vitamin A. At the lowest dose the animal is clearly deficient and loses vision, which is a sign of vitamin A deficiency. As the dose increases, visual ability returns. With a higher intake the liver, which stores vitamin A, has minimal storage so most of the vitamin A is being used. Theoretically this is where the RDA might be set. But at even higher doses vitamin A stores in the liver reach maximum. This is the beginning of the Optimum Range. At even higher doses, maximum production of young is reached. If one were to continue this graph the vitamin would eventually become toxic. What is interesting to note is that the amount of vitamin A needed to produce maximum young was 430 iu per kg of body mass. In a 9 st woman this would be equivalent to 27,500 iu, somewhat higher than the RDA of 2,250 iu.

ARE YOU GETTING ENOUGH?

The majority of people don't even get the RDA of these essential nutrients. What's more, a lot of essential nutrients don't even have RDAs. For example, the pregnant woman needs 20 mg per day of zinc, yet in Britain there is no RDA. The average woman gets up to 10 mg only. Zinc levels in breast milk steadily decline showing a negative zinc balance. 73 per cent of women don't get as much as 500 mg of calcium yet the pregnant woman needs 1,200 mg. In fact, we estimate that only five in a hundred women during pregnancy have a diet that meets all the basic nutrient allowances. This is why supplementation is not only a wise precaution but is in my opinion a definite must in pregnancy. To be able to approach optimum nutrition during pregnancy it is necessary not only to have a good diet but to supplement additional nutrients. The next chapter explains how.

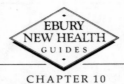

CHAPTER 10

SUPERNUTRITION FOR A HEALTHY PREGNANCY

SOME doctors wrongly warn against vitamin and mineral supplementation during pregnancy. Among those who are unfamiliar with nutrition there is a belief that one needs be extremely careful with pregnant women and children. This of course is true; however, the best care possible is to ensure adequate nutrient intake and to minimize exposure to pollutants and unnecessary medication.

It is well established that nutritional deficiency in animals will cause birth abnormalities. This has been shown with B2 (riboflavin), B3 (niacin), B5 (pantothenic acid), B6 (pyridoxine) and folic acid. In fact, if you are in the process of improving your nutrition it is better to wait a few months before getting pregnant. According to Dr Carl Pfeiffer (1) 'Pregnancy is a severe nutritional stress. Ideally, good nutrition should begin many years before pregnancy.' Many illnesses, including flu and the common cold, delay conception, probably because of the depletion of nutrients that these circumstances cause. It is also best to wait till these have passed before trying to conceive.

To ensure optimum nutrition in pregnancy it is necessary to take some vitamin and mineral supplements even if your diet is well balanced. However, there are some vitamins which should not be taken in large amounts during pregnancy. One of these is vitamin A.

THE DANGERS OF TAKING TOO MUCH VITAMIN A

Vitamin A is a fat-soluble vitamin found in foods of animal origin and particularly in liver, since this is where it is stored in the body. Cod liver oil is a popular source for vitamin A although it can also be made synthetically. Some synthetic forms of vitamin A are far more toxic than the natural vitamin A and it is these that have caused great concern recently. Reporting in the *Lancet*, TV reporter Joan Shenton had this to say about vitamin A (2): 'The programmes featured two published cases of hypervitaminosis. One woman took excessive amounts of vitamin A to enhance her suntan and maintain the health of skin, hair, nails and eyes. She suffered (among other things) extensive desquamation of the skin, and almost complete loss of body hair (3). A man who took low levels of vitamin A for acne had bifrontal headache, abdominal pain, severe weight loss and desquamation of the skin (4). We also featured three "health food" supplements which were tablets or capsules of 25,000 iu of vitamin A freely available in Britain.'

This report sounds sensible but highlights three common misunderstandings about vitamin A. The first is that all forms of vitamin A are toxic. This is not true. The second, that doses of 25,000 iu of natural vitamin A are toxic. There is no evidence to support this. And the third point so commonly missed is that vitamins become more toxic if given on their own without a proper balance of the other nutrients with which they work.

Firstly, it is only a particular form of vitamin A, isotretinoin (Accutane) which appears so toxic. It has been marketed as a supplement for treating acne and has an 'X' rating for use in pregnancy (5). According to a report in the *Journal of the American Academy of Dermatologists* (skin specialists) 'It is this (isotretinoin) form we need to watch out for. Other forms of vitamin A don't appear to be nearly so toxic according to the American Food and Drug Administration' (6).

Since any substance, even water, is potentially toxic how much is too much? Naturopath Leon Chaitow, writing in the *Journal of Alternative Medicine*, says 'Levels below 500,000 iu are not thought to carry the risk but caution is urged.' That's a far cry from the doses of 4,500 iu up to 25,000 iu found in some vitamin A supplements. He also points out that the teratogenicity of vitamin A is compounded by other nutrient imbalances, particularly choline and vitamin E deficiencies.

Vitamin A is vital for proper foetal growth and plays an important part in visual development. The RDA for pregnant women is 2,250 iu and the optimum level anywhere between 7,500 iu and 15,000 iu. However, in the view of the somewhat unfounded reports of vitamin A toxicity it is wise not to supplement any more than this, unless you have clear deficiency symptoms and are under the supervision of a doctor or nutritionist.

VITAMIN D IS VITAL FOR HEALTHY BONES

Unlike any other vitamin, vitamin D can be made in the skin in the presence of sunlight. Vitamin D deficiency is not common in Britain, except in pregnant Asian women, who, for reasons of skin colour, filter out the sun's ultraviolet rays and produce less vitamin D. However, although vitamin D deficiency is not good news for the mother, some evidence suggests that the baby is not greatly affected. In a study reported in the *British Medical Journal*, the babies of 45 Asian women, 19 of whom had received supplements of 1,000 iu of vitamin D, and 12 white women were compared for mineralization of bones. None of the children showed any abnormal level of bone mineralization (7).

Vitamin D is found with vitamin A in animal produce and in liver; it is also high in milk. Although there is no RDA for vitamin D as such, the recommended daily level is 400 iu.

VITAMIN K AND CAULIFLOWER

Vitamin K is called the clotting factor because it is involved in the manufacture of prothrombin, which makes your blood clot. Normally it is manufactured by bacteria in the gut. However, a baby's gut is sterile after birth and must rely on the mother's supply. Breast milk contains a factor that inhibits vitamin K so breast-feeding mothers need to take special care to eat enough cauliflower and cabbage which are high in vitamin K. Although very rare, unexplained bleeding in young infants can be due to vitamin K deficiency.

THE B COMPLEX VITAMINS

Many individual nutrients make up the B Complex group. These include B1, B2, B3, B5, B6, B12, folic acid, biotin and PABA. Although choline and inositol are not strictly vitamins since they can be made by the body, they are often included in the B Complex group because a greater dietary supply can enhance health.

B1 – Thiamine

Thiamine is known as the 'morale vitamin' because of its role in balancing the nervous system and its link with improved learning capacity. It is vital for proper utilization of carbohydrates, but other than that it has no particular role to play in pregnancy.

B2 – Riboflavin

Riboflavin is one vitamin which appears to have no extra benefit in large amounts during pregnancy. In fact, great excesses of B2 may have a detrimental effect on birthweight. However, a large proportion of pregnant women (40 per cent) do become deficient in B2 by the end of pregnancy (9). A study on Kenyan women revealed that B2 levels were low in the blood of 73 per cent of women tested, although no deficiency was present in the placenta. These researchers found there was a correlation between mothers with low B2 and low birthweight children. This study also found that B1 was deficient in 59 per cent of the mothers and 15 per cent of the placentas; B6 was deficient in 35 per cent of the mothers and 24 per cent of the placentas (10). So as far as B2 is concerned getting a basic level of 25 mg a day is totally adequate.

B3 – Nicotinic Acid, Niacin

The needs for vitamin B3 go up in pregnancy. It has many functions to perform. Perhaps most important of all, B3 is a precursor for serotonin, an important nerve transmitter involved in maintaining good sleep patterns. It also makes the blood vessels dilate and helps get oxygen to every cell in the body. The RDA for a pregnant woman is 18 mg although the optimum intake is more like 50 mg a day.

B5 – Pantothenic Acid

The word pantothenic acid comes from the Greek word 'pantos' meaning everywhere, because it is found in every living cell both in your food and in your body. It is vital for making acetylcholine which is a chemical involved in memory and is involved in many enzyme systems in the body. There is no RDA, but the optimum daily intake is 50 mg.

B6

Britain has no recommended levels for B6. In America 2 mg is recommended daily, and extrapolated from this figure (based on a pregnant woman's increased need for protein, which B6 helps to metabolize) the RDA for a pregnant woman is 2.6 mg. But this simply isn't enough to maintain normal biochemical functions. B6 levels in the blood decline rapidly during pregnancy dropping from 11.3 mcg/ml to 3 mcg/ml by the end, strongly implying B6 depletion. Studies have also shown decreased B6 dependent enzyme activity until people are given at least 7.5 mg on top of the average deficient diet which supplies less than 1.5 mg (11). So that's 9 mg in all just to prevent obvious deficiency. The optimum level for B6 is probably between 25 and 100 mg, and more likely 50 to 100 mg during pregnancy and breast feeding.

B12 and Folic Acid

Vitamin B12 and folic acid are particularly important in pregnancy. Normal foetal development depends upon these nutrients. One of the indications of the importance of B12 is the fact that the levels found in new-born babies are more than twice that found in the mother. Adequate B12 nutrition also appears to increase the uptake of folic acid. In one study in which pregnant women were supplemented with B12, folic acid levels in the mother's blood rose significantly (12).

The (US) RDA for folic acid is 800 mcg during pregnancy. The average intake is about 200 mcg, so the average woman falls a long way short of what is needed. In fact, the World Health Organization reports that from one-half to one-third of expectant mothers suffer from folic acid deficiency in the last three months of pregnancy (13). Folic acid in food can be lost by storing or cooking. Folic acid is needed to manufacture DNA and with B12 helps to make red blood cells. Folic acid deficiency can produce irritability, sluggishness, forgetfulness and cheilosis (a condition characterized by lesions at the side of the mouth) (14). But the most significant symptom of deficiency in pregnancy is pernicious anaemia. According to Dr Pfeiffer 'Many women with a history of abortion and miscarriage have been able to complete successful childbirth subsequent to folic acid supplementation' (15).

It is now generally thought that a folic acid supplement of at least 300 mcg should be taken to minimize the risk of deficiency.

Biotin

This vital B vitamin is often excluded in popular A to Zs of vitamins, yet its role in pregnancy is of the greatest importance. Biotin is needed to make fatty acids and, most of all, is needed to ensure that B12 and folic acid are used properly. The normal recommended intake is 150 mcg to 300 mcg. Probably 300 mcg represents an ideal intake during pregnancy.

Biotin can be made by the bacteria in the gut. Deficiency is extremely rare and occurs primarily in those with digestive disorders. One word of caution if you eat raw eggs! These contain avidin which prevents the absorption of biotin.

VITAMIN C

Vitamin C has so many roles in pregnancy it's hard to know where to start. It helps make collagen, the intercellular glue that keeps skin supple, and is therefore vital for preventing stretch marks. It helps to carry oxygen to every cell, nourishing the baby, and builds a strong infection-fighting system, keeping the mother in good form. Its need goes up in pregnancy and a daily intake of 2,000 mg is recommended.

VITAMIN E

Like vitamin C, E helps get oxygen to the cells and protects the vital RNA and DNA from damage which could result in congenital defects for the baby. It also speeds up wound healing and helps to keep skin supple. It is particularly useful if applied externally for those who give birth by Caesarian section. I have seen scars completely disappear with application of vitamin E. The optimum level in pregnancy is 400 iu per day.

MINERALS FOR THE HEALTHY MOTHER

Just as important as vitamins, and perhaps even more frequently deficient, are the trace minerals. 'Trace element deficiencies and imbalances due to a multitude of causes may be an underlying problem in many cases of neonatal death, congenital anomaly and disorders of pregnancy, as well as poor childhood development' according to nutritionist Elizabeth Lodge Rees writing in *Trace Elements in Health* (Butterworth, England). While we are very aware of the need for extra iron, what about the lesser-known trace elements zinc, manganese, chromium or selenium?

TOO MANY IRONS IN THE FIRE

Iron deficiency is very common in pregnancy. As many as 32 per cent of women may show mild iron deficiency anaemia in pregnancy, with symptoms of lethargy, pale skin and a sore tongue. For this reason doctors always test the haemoglobin level in the blood. Haemoglobin is a protein containing iron that carries oxygen to every cell in the body. Haemoglobin levels frequently fall below 12.6 g/dl at which point some iron should be supplemented or, if the diet is low, this should be corrected.

The RDA for iron is 12 mg in the UK and 18 mg in the USA. Rarely more than 25 mg is needed. However, pregnant women are often prescribed 180 mg or more. This is far too much and interferes with the absorption of other minerals. In fact, one study compared the effect of supplementing 200 to 300 mg of ferrous sulphate, which supplied 60 mg to 90 mg of iron to 300 pregnant women. The rise in haemoglobin was no more in those taking 300 mg compared to those taking 200 mg, making the larger dose redundant. Iron absorption is considerably enhanced by vitamin C so eating vitamin C rich foods helps. By having a glass of orange with your boiled egg you can increase iron absorption four-fold. Vitamin B2 also helps absorb iron (16).

There is no doubt, however, that iron is needed in larger amounts during pregnancy and childhood. 20 to 30 mg of iron is quite sufficient. Many doctors still prescribe 60 mg or more to pregnant women. Except in cases where there has been excessive blood loss this much simply isn't necessary (17).

CALCIUM AND MAGNESIUM – NATURE'S TRANQUILLIZERS

Calcium, phosphorus and magnesium, found in bone, are the major minerals in the human body. A pregnant woman needs a lot more than usual for the baby to build healthy bones; calcium and magnesium also play a vital role in nerve and muscle cell maintenance. When they are deficient, muscle cramps and tremors can occur and the nervous system can become 'out of tune'. Magnesium, particularly, has a calming effect on the nerves.

The normal requirement for calcium is 500 mg. In a survey released in 1986, it was found that 73 per cent of women get less than 500 mg of calcium. The requirement for calcium in pregnancy is 1,200 mg per day. That's almost three times more than the average intake and quite frankly it's just about impossible to get without supplementing. Green leafy vegetables, nuts and seeds are high in calcium and magnesium. Many diet textbooks recommend mothers to drink half a litre of milk which supplies 600 mg of calcium, but no magnesium.

Dolomite is the best way of supplementing calcium since it contains magnesium in the right balance. Some dolomite supplements contain extra vitamin D, which is needed to ensure proper absorption of calcium.

Zinc is so important in pregnancy that a whole chapter has been devoted to it. A pregnant woman needs at least 20 mg a day and frequently gets less than half of this from her diet. There are more grounds for supplementing zinc in pregnancy than any other mineral.

Zinc and copper are well-known enemies so zinc needs go up if copper is in excess. Although copper levels rise in pregnancy and too much can be dangerous, too little is not a good idea either. A good wholefood diet with plenty of beans and lentils will provide enough copper. If supplements are taken, no more than 1 mg a day should be taken.

THE MYSTERIOUS MINERALS – CHROMIUM, SELENIUM AND MANGANESE

Very little is known about the role of trace elements chromium, selenium and manganese in pregnancy. One study investigated manganese levels in mother and baby, comparing these levels to premature births and to congenital malformations. They found that infants and mothers of infants with congenital malformations had lower hair manganese levels than those pre-term and full-term infants and mothers (19). Manganese is commonly deficient in Britain and particularly so in people on a junk-food diet.

Chromium is needed to make Glucose Tolerance Factor (GTF) which helps to lower blood sugar level by carrying blood glucose to the cells where it can be used or stored. The average person gets anywhere between 8 and 89 mcg per day from diet. The guidelines for daily intake are 50 to 250 mcg. Chromium may well be deficient, especially in those with a high-sugar diet. In animals, chromium deficiency slows growth.

Selenium has been called the anti-cancer element because of its vital role in protecting cells from harmful oxides. Like vitamin A it is toxic in large amounts; however, anything up to 150 mcg can be supplemented without danger. It is commonly deficient in the British diet.

SUPPLEMENTS FOR A HEALTHY PREGNANCY

The chart on page 72 shows the Optimum Levels of nutrients in pregnancy that we work to at the Institute for Optimum Nutrition. Some of these are the same as the RDAs and some are a lot higher. All are based on our experiences and current medical research. The Optimum Dietary Intake column shows the levels that an optimum diet could supply. The final column 'Minimum Supplemental Level' represents what one would need to supplement to reach the Optimum Levels, given that you are eating a well-balanced diet.

But don't worry. You don't have to take hundreds of different vitamin pills. All these can be provided in three or four supplements provided you choose your formulas carefully. The best formula available is the Pregnancy Pack by Health + Plus which is based on our calculations. Other good vitamin companies include Healthcrafts, Nature's Best, Cantassium, Natural Flow and Meadowcroft, all of whom have good multivitamins and minerals which can meet a substantial part of your needs from this table.

Nutrient	Optimum Level	Optimum Dietary Intake	Minimum Supplemental Level
Vitamins			
A	7,500 iu	25,000 iu	(max 7,500 iu)
D	400 iu	200 iu	200 iu
E	400 iu	20 iu	380 iu
C	1,500 mg	200 mg	1,300 mg
B1 (thiamine)	25 mg	2 mg	23 mg
B2 (riboflavin)	25 mg	3 mg	22 mg
B3 (niacin)	50 mg	25 mg	25 mg
B5 (pantothenic acid)	50 mg	30 mg	20 mg
B6 (pyridoxine)	100 mg	21 mg	79 mg
B12	50 mcg	15 mcg	35 mcg
Folic Acid	800 mcg	600 mcg	200 mcg
Biotin	200 mcg	100 mcg	100 mcg
Minerals			
Sodium	3,000 mg	2,000 mg	–
Potassium	5,000 mg	6,000 mg	–
Calcium	1,200 mg	1,500 mg	(max 800 mg)
Magnesium	600 mg	600 mg	(max 300 mg)
Iron	18 mg	25 mg	(max 20 mg)
Zinc	20 mg	10 mg	10 mg
Chromium	50 mcg	?30 mcg	20 mcg
Manganese	5 mg	?3 mg	2 mg
Selenium	25 mcg	?15 mcg	10 mcg

Insufficient data is available for those nutrients marked ?

HOW TO TAKE SUPPLEMENTS

Supplements are best absorbed if taken with a meal. Some people prefer to take dolomite in the evening as this has a calming effect. B vitamins and vitamin C often have an energizing effect and are best taken in the morning. These are also better absorbed if the dosage is spread throughout the day. So, for example, it would be better to take 1,000 mg of vitamin C with breakfast and 1,000 mg of vitamin C with lunch. However, if taking them twice or three times a day would mean you'd almost certainly forget to take some of them then it's better to take the whole lot together.

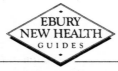

CHAPTER 11

AFTER-BIRTH BOOSTERS

G IVING birth is hard work and the chances are you will be very tired afterwards. There are some people who get an after-birth 'high'. If this is the case I strongly suggest following a similar regime as for exhausted mums – the help you get from new grannies, uncles, aunts and friends may not be offered so readily again. Also you will need all your energy for the inevitable few weeks of sleepless nights.

If you are in hospital you may well want to leave as soon as possible as it will be very hard to eat healthily. The other babies will probably keep you awake and, depending on the hospital's policies and the thoughts of the individual nurses, you may well find it difficult to completely demand feed your baby (more on this in the next chapter). Please remember that if you are going to go home you will need help when you get there. It could be very miserable being at home with a new-born if your husband has gone off to work, leaving you to worry alone about how often you should change the baby's nappy and whether demand feeding really means feeding the baby every 30 minutes! You will also need support when your milk comes in (about day five) and waving goodbye to a husband off to work could reduce you to floods of tears.

If you do decide to stay in hospital for a few days, see if you can arrange for a relative or friend to bring in vitality packed salads, a nourishing nut roast, a baked potato filled with cheese from the local takeaway, a loaf of wholemeal bread and a jar of peanut butter, some muesli and lots of fruit. Vegetarians often seem to get better food in hospitals, so even if you normally eat meat it is worth saying you are vegetarian. Don't be afraid of stating your likes and dislikes regarding hospital food. After all, hospitals do not serve Jewish people bacon due to their beliefs so why should they serve you plastic bread, greasy chips and over-cooked vegetables?

When you arrive home or if you have your baby at home, do not be tempted to rush about tidying up and doing lots of cooking. Ask a helper to scrub a whole 5 lb bag of potatoes. These can later be put straight in the oven and baked. If people come round to see the baby and want to stay to eat, ask them to cook the dinner or send them out on shopping errands – they will love to feel useful.

Don't forget that your most important task is to ensure a plentiful milk supply for your baby and to do this you will need plenty of rest and enough food, especially if you have not gained any extra weight during your pregnancy. Start getting into the habit of having daytime naps as broken nights are not nearly as rejuvenating as complete ones.

BEATING THE BABY BLUES

It is not uncommon for new mothers to suffer from depression immediately after the birth. A small percentage become psychotic, completely out of touch with reality. No doubt there is a psychological component to consider. Now you have a baby – a big responsibility – and there's nothing you can do about it. However, many researchers believe that this post-natal depression is brought on by hormonal and chemical changes which can be stopped with good nutrition.

THE COPPER CONNECTION

During pregnancy copper levels continue to rise, reaching a peak after the birth. Copper levels can be kept in hand by adequate zinc status. As already explained, many women are zinc deficient causing a further increase in copper. During the birth itself substantial amounts of zinc are lost as zinc is rapidly depleted in any stress or profound physical event. Giving birth is both of these. For women who give birth by Caesarian section, zinc is used up because zinc is involved in wound healing and rapidly concentrates in any injured area.

The net consequence of this is that copper is extremely high and zinc extremely low straight after the birth. This imbalance is known outside of pregnancy to be connected with psychosis and depression. Dr Carl Pfeiffer, the world's foremost authority on zinc, copper and the brain, says 'We have never seen post-natal depression or psychosis in any of our patients treated with zinc and B6.'

SPECIAL NUTRIENT NEEDS FOR TWO SPECIAL PEOPLE

But zinc isn't the only nutrient you'll be needing after giving birth. The placenta is rich in minerals which are all lost from the body after birth. Our ancestors used to eat the placenta providing these minerals and some primitive tribes still keep up this practice. While some people advocate 'placenta stew' I'd much rather have a multi-mineral supplement!

The most important minerals are iron, which may have been significantly lost depending on the degree of bleeding at birth, calcium and magnesium, because these are essential for energy production during labour and will be needed in large amounts for the breast-feeding baby, and finally zinc and manganese.

The vitality vitamins are the same old favourites. Plenty of B Complex, especially B6, B12 and folic acid. Also vitamin C which is rapidly used up during the birth. Particularly important are vitamins A, D and E. Vitamin A is vital for any bruising and wound healing and will help restore your abdomen, uterus and vagina to their former size. Vitamin E is also very beneficial for bruising and wound healing, but most of all, together with vitamin C, encourages skin elasticity and the contraction of skin across the abdomen. If you have had any stretch marks (which you shouldn't have if you are getting enough zinc) vitamin E will help to reduce these. It should be applied externally, using a 1,000 iu vitamin E capsule and rubbing this into the skin. Alternatively you can use a strong vitamin E cream.

It takes many months for the abdomen to return to normal and for many women it never does. Exercise and good nutrition make all the difference but don't expect instant results. The same is true for the vagina and uterus. This area can be extremely sensitive for many months, especially in women who have an episiotomy or who tear during the birth. For the vast majority this means they will have little desire for sex and intercourse may be painful.

THE AFTER-BIRTH BOOSTERS

Supplement	AM	PM
Multivite	1	
B Complex (with B12 10 mcg)	1	
B6 100 mg and Zinc 10 mg	1	1
Folic Acid 800 mcg	1	
C 1,000 mg	1	1
A and D 10,000 iu		1
E 1,000 iu	1	
Multi Mins (with Iron 12 mg)		1
Dolomite		1

So here's our after-birth booster supplement programme to turn you into a supermum. This programme (see page 75) is designed for the first two weeks only. Since you'll have enough on your plate without running around trying to find supplements of B6 and zinc, I recommend you pack up this programme into daily envelopes and if you are going into hospital take a few of these with you.

WHY BREAST-FEEDING MUMS NEED VITAMIN K

The risk for vitamin K deficiency in your baby after birth is higher in breast-fed babies. This fat-soluble vitamin is needed for proper blood clotting and, if deficient, bleeding can occur. It is not at all common, but can occur in the young infant up to four weeks old. There are two reasons for this. Firstly, fat-soluble substances are not so readily transferred from mother to baby via the placenta and most new-born babies have only a third as much of the vitamin K dependent clotting factors in their blood at birth. So they need to get some from their milk. Breast milk contains only 1 or 2 mcg per dl, compared to cow's milk which contains 5 to 17 mcg per dl. The baby needs about 5 mcg per day. Foods such as cauliflower and cabbage are particularly high in vitamin K and should be eaten by the breast-feeding mother.

The other reason that vitamin K deficiency can develop is that normally it is synthesized by bacteria in the gut. However, a new-born baby's gut is sterile for the first few days of life. Breast milk is also sterile and doesn't encourage the vitamin K producing bacteria to flourish. So the baby is dependent on the mother eating plenty of vegetables, especially cabbage and cauliflower.

As far as the rest of your diet is concerned make sure you eat well in the days preceding the birth. For the birth itself be sure to have drinks with sweetness or honey in them. Fruit juices or herb teas with honey are best. It's important to keep your supply of 'fuel' topped up. Some women run out of energy and end up breaking down body protein and getting too many ketones in the blood, which are the by-product of using protein for energy. This is a primary cause for an elongated labour.

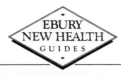

CHAPTER 12

BREAST IS BEST

S EVENTY years ago this chapter would not have been needed, as breast feeding was the norm. However, the number of women who choose to breast feed has declined so much that now women have to be persuaded back into it. There are many advantages to breast feeding, the most important one being nutritional. Although we have advanced slightly from the days when cow's milk was boiled, diluted and had sugar added to it, we have still not produced a formula milk that is identical to human milk.

Formulas do not contain selenium, important for the prevention of heart disease and cancer, or chromium, needed to produce the glucose tolerance factor. The manganese in breast milk is 20 times more absorbable than that in formula milk (1) and iron is also more absorbable. Formulas for tiny babies are sweetened with lactose, as is breast milk; however, once a baby is over four months old the sweetener used is corn syrup. This will provide glucose which is a much more readily absorbable form of sugar.

Different milks from different mammals vary enormously. For instance, whale milk is so high in fat (and calories) that it resembles double cream. This enables the baby whale to develop a thick layer of blubber to protect it from the cold sea. The initial reasons for giving babies cow's milk half a century ago are very dubious, as, in fact, donkey's milk resembles human milk far more closely. Cows were, however, much more available and produce more milk.

Once feeding is established breast feeding is far more convenient than messing around with bottles. The baby is far less likely to get gastro-enteritis and the risk of developing an allergy to cow's milk is reduced as the baby's gut will leak whole cow's milk molecules. Many women think they will not be able to produce enough milk as their breasts are too small. However, the increase in size during pregnancy is far more indicative of ability to produce milk than original size, also the change from a breast-feeding culture to one that predominantly does not breast feed in the space of two generations is too fast to genetically affect the ability to lactate. Nearly all the cases of inadequate milk supply are due to inadequate teaching and/or social embarrassment.

This chapter doesn't aim to teach you how to breast feed: what you can and should do is contact your local breast-feeding group, for instance the National Childbirth Trust or La Leche League. However, there are some guidelines, and these are given below.

HOW OFTEN SHOULD YOU FEED YOUR BABY?

If you let your baby feed whenever she wants to (including at night) you are far more likely to get a good supply going without engorgement or sore nipples. A study done on African women sleeping with their small babies showed that new-born babies went for a maximum of 20 minutes between feeds. Having your baby in your bed, at least for the first few weeks, is a good way to get the milk going. This also has the advantage of you not having to worry about keeping her warm at night. It has been shown that less than five feeds a day will not keep an adequate milk supply going, so if you feel like you are constantly feeding your baby you are probably doing the right thing! As a hangover from bottle feeding where the amount the baby receives is a carefully measured amount, people started recommending noting, and restricting, the sucking time at each breast, despite the fact that different babies suck at different strengths (some are plain greedy). It is impossible to overfeed a breast-fed baby and so long as the baby is growing (even if slowly) everything will be all right.

LOOKING AFTER YOURSELF

It is, however, important to look after yourself. This means getting adequate nutrient levels, particularly zinc and the B vitamins, eating a good diet, eating enough (for someone who has not gained any extra weight during pregnancy this may mean eating enormous amounts) and getting enough rest. The baby that is on the breast constantly all through the evening is probably not getting what he needs due to you overdoing it during the day and early evening. In a study (2) it was shown that supplementing the diet with protein increased the milk supply and consequently the size of the babies. It is important to ensure an adequate protein intake, particularly if you are not eating meat. It is a good idea to set it up so that you can have healthy snacks throughout the day. This will mean plenty of wholemeal bread with peanut butter, sugar-free jam, honey or a tofu, tahini, soya sauce combination, yoghurt with banana, muesli with fruit, apple and cheese, dried fruits and nuts and plenty of fresh fruit (contrary to popular belief breast feeding will probably end up more expensive than bottle feeding if you and your baby are optimumly nourished). If you have gained weight during your pregnancy you will still need to give yourself maximum nourishment and this will mean eating lots of fruit and plenty of fresh salads.

Getting enough liquid is just as important as getting enough food. Your baby will be taking between one and two pints of water through your breast milk which needs to be replaced. Including your normal daily drinks you could be drinking as much as six pints of liquid a day. As most substances cross into your breast milk in varying degrees of concentration, it is important not to drink tea, coffee, chocolate, cola drinks or any other drink containing sugar or artificial additives. Choose healthy alternatives like herb teas, coffee substitutes (available from health food shops), fruit juice diluted half and half with water, sparkling mineral water and just plain humble water. If you are drinking enough you should not have to give your baby extra water or fruit juice. The only time you should give extra water is under the doctor's advice if your baby is constipated, has a fever, diarrhoea or is vomiting. Breast milk really is a complete food for your baby.

Breast milk is usually a bluey-white colour. But mothers on vitamin supplements have milk that is distinctly yellow and more like cow's milk in appearance. Could it be that we are giving cows better nutrition than ourselves? This yellow hue is in part caused by sufficient levels of B2 and beta-carotene, the vegetable form of vitamin A.

THE PROS AND CONS OF BREAST FEEDING

There are many more advantages than disadvantages to breast feeding. For example, during the first, vital weeks of life your baby's main protection against disease is obtained from the anti-bodies found in breast milk – these are not put in formula milk. There is even some evidence that the incidence of cot deaths is higher among bottle-fed babies, particularly during the time of change between breast and bottle. However, it is not known why. Breast milk is easier to digest and this could be a contributing factor.

Sucking on a breast is also much harder work than sucking on a bottle. So breast-fed babies develop a much stronger jaw, which stands them in good stead for later on when they starts eating salads.

BREAST FEEDING IS NATURE'S CONTRACEPTIVE

The last thing you'll want to do while looking after a hungry baby is get pregnant. As long as you're breast feeding there's little chance of that since the high circulating level of the hormone prolactin prevents ovulation and menstruation making the breast-feeding mother temporarily infertile. Once you stop or reduce breast feeding substantially the return to ovulation is faster if your diet is good. However, please note that breast feeding alone is not a one hundred per cent reliable form of contraception (3).

WHY BREAST FEEDING HELPS YOU TO LOSE WEIGHT

On the right diet many women find they lose weight while breast feeding without any risk of poor nourishment for themselves or their babies. While the US RDA for a lactating woman is 2,750 kcal, in one study 45 lactating women on a 2,186 calorie diet remained perfectly healthy, full of energy and produced sufficient breast milk. Their weight after four months dropped by a little over 11 pounds. Their babies grew just as fast as those of other mothers whose calorie intake was higher. Provided the quality of food is good, losing weight during lactation is compatible with successful breast feeding (4).

BREAST FEEDING DOESN'T GUARANTEE
GOOD NUTRITION

However, mother's milk is only as good as the mother. And most mothers' nutrition is not good enough to guarantee the baby the best start in life. For instance, take vitamin B6 levels in milk. An infant needs 0.3 mg per day according to the US recommended daily allowance. A group of women whose diets were analysed to contain on average 1.8 mg a day, which is marginally below the RDA of 2 mg, were given varying levels of B6 supplementation, from nothing up to 20 mg, which is 10 times higher than the RDA. The levels of B6 found in breast milk provided the equivalent of 0.06 mg for those unsupplemented, up to 0.28 mg for those supplementing an extra 20 mg a day. In other words, even this level of supplementation didn't meet the baby's basic needs for B6. Supplements of 50 mg of B6 are recommended in pregnancy to reach optimal levels. However, a word of caution. Doses in excess of 200 to 600 mg a day have been reported to suppress lactation. There is no danger of this at the 50 mg level (5).

However, not all B vitamins need to be supplemented in such relatively large amounts. Provided folic acid is supplemented during pregnancy it appears likely that breast-fed babies will be getting enough.

BABIES DON'T BECOME 'VITAMIN DEPENDENT'

Although some people mistakenly feel that taking large amounts of vitamin C might somehow pass on a vitamin C dependency to the new-born baby, unlike vitamin B6, there appears to be a mechanism that stops the baby getting more than it needs. The breast milk of mothers supplementing 1,000 mg or more of vitamin C provides between 40 mg and 86 mg daily for the infant. Taking more vitamin C didn't increase the level in breast milk although the mother's excretion of vitamin C did increase (7). So at least as far as the baby is concerned 1,000 mg of vitamin C a day is adequate for the mother.

BREAST MILK IS BETTER FOR FAT-SOLUBLE VITAMINS

Vitamin E is one vitamin that comes out on top in breast milk. Normally at least 0.6 mg/g of vitamin E in total lipids in serum is considered adequate for the infant. In one Brazilian study only one in 176 breast-fed children had less than this, compared to over half in the group that were fed on cow's milk only. Although no signs of deficiency occurred in those with inadequate vitamin E status, babies fed predominantly on cow's milk should have a little extra E (8).

Another study has shown that breast milk is higher in vitamin D than ordinary milk. The researchers also identified a particular kind of vitamin D called 25-OHD, which has been shown to be 2.5 times more effective for preventing rickets, indicating its more potent effect on increasing calcium utilization. Vitamin D helps to increase calcium supply in the baby by encouraging the absorption of calcium from the gut. This special form of vitamin D is naturally present in breast milk. The suggestion from this research is that this more active form of vitamin D should be added to infant formulas (9).

BREAST MILK IS ZINC DEFICIENT

A new-born infant up to six months needs 3 mg of zinc a day. Yet the average amount supplied daily in human milk is only 1.3 mg during the first three months and even less, only 0.6 mg a day, in the last three months of breast feeding. This indicates just how hard it is to provide adequate zinc for the baby. Mothers and babies alike become increasingly deficient as breast feeding continues. This conclusion has been confirmed in a study that investigated the effects on zinc status of 16 nursing mothers and the weight and zinc excretion of their exclusively breast-fed babies. Those with lower birthweight babies had low serum levels of zinc and the babies tended to excrete less zinc, presumably indicating a greater need (10).

However, breast-milk zinc is generally far better absorbed than dietary zinc, so these low figures may not be as bad as they seem. It may well be the breast-feeding mother who suffers more from slight zinc deficiency than the baby (11). The biggest danger to zinc supply to the baby is prolonged breast feeding when the mother is on an inadequate diet. Research has clearly shown that breast milk concentrations drop substantially throughout breast feeding to well below 50 per cent of the recommended daily intake for infants (12). There is little doubt that a breast-feeding mother needs to get at least 25 mg of zinc a day, and that means supplementing at least 15 mg.

SELENIUM AND BREAST MILK

Selenium is another mineral that is needed in greater amounts during pregnancy. Some countries, like Finland, have poor soil levels of selenium and poor dietary intakes. Studies on Finnish women have shown clearly that on a diet containing 30 mcg of selenium a day, breast milk levels of selenium decline as breast feeding continues, and that higher dietary intake increases breast milk levels. Studies of selenium levels in placenta and amniotic tissue show levels three times higher than those in the mother's blood. The suggestion here is that selenium deficiency for the baby is avoided at all costs during pregnancy, including depriving the mother of this essential nutrient (14). The intake of selenium in Britain is around 60 mcg, although a significant number of people get less than 30 mcg a day. The suggested daily intake for selenium, which has no RDA in Britain, is 50 to 200 mcg. A daily supplement of 50 mcg is recommended during lactation.

WHICH FORMULAS ARE BEST?

Not all women have the choice whether or not to breast feed their babies. So which formula is best? Rather than list the many different makes, it's better to know what to look for. Firstly you'll want to avoid formulas that contain added sugar, glucose or corn syrup. It simply isn't needed. Then it's a matter of comparing nutrient content. Probably the easiest way to pick out a good formula milk is to compare the zinc content. It should also contain manganese, chromium and selenium although many don't. In America the amino acid taurine, now thought to be essential for babies, is often added.

There are a number of myths about formula milks. The manufacturers will try to tell you that you need to change formulas once a baby is three months old. This is totally unnecessary. It is far better to choose your formula and stick to it. Some mothers make a more concentrated solution than instructed because they think the milk looks too thin. This is wrong. Breast milk is thin but nutritious stuff. More doesn't mean better. Labelling and advertising emphasize the vitamin and mineral content of formula milks. However, they are by law required to contain certain levels of these nutrients. Sadly, it is assumed that all mothers give their babies vitamin drops provided by the DHSS free of charge. So formulas don't even have to supply the RDA for nutrients. Check the figures carefully.

IS GOAT'S MILK BETTER THAN COW'S MILK?

Goat's milk is thought to be less allergenic than cow's milk, and some people recommend it instead of cow's milk for baby food. But goat's milk is not ideal on a number of counts. Firstly, most goat's milk is unpasteurized and the risk of infection for a child up to one year is simply not worth it. Secondly, like cow's milk, the concentrations of folic acid, vitamin C and D are too low. From the nutritional point of view it is little different from cow's milk. However, some goat's milk is less contaminated with drugs, and if boiled or pasteurized and obtained from animals tested for brucellosis or tuberculosis it is perfectly safe.

Another alternative used in formula milks for children with milk allergy is soya milk. Soya has often been criticized for its poor absorbable zinc. This was thought to be due to the presence of phytate which inhibits zinc uptake. However, it may be the high iron content, not the phytate, that competes with zinc. Studies have shown that when twice as much iron as zinc is eaten, this inhibits zinc. Soya formulas contain much more iron than zinc, because even more is added to these formulas. Infants consuming iron-enriched soya formulas do have lower zinc levels. The ideal zinc/iron ratio in breast milk and presumably in diet is around 1:1.

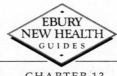

CHAPTER 13

WEANING – WHEN AND WHAT

THE question 'when to wean' is hard to answer. The question 'when not to wean' is easier. To start with, no two babies are the same so no two babies will be weaned at the same time. There is no set age or weight at which to wean a baby. Penelope Leach, in her book *Baby and Child*, calculates that a 12 lb baby can no longer be totally breast fed. I personally totally breast fed my baby until he was over 20 lb – as did many of my friends. After all, my son Kyle was 12 lb by the time he was four weeks old and that's certainly too soon to stop breast feeding.

WEANING FALLACIES

This advice to stop breast feeding when the baby is 12 lb is based on some erroneous assumptions. First, they calculate how many calories a baby needs in a 24-hour period, working on the assumption that a baby's stomach can hold about 7 or 8 fl oz and that the baby will have only five feeds in a day. 35 fl oz provides only enough calories for a 12 lb baby. What Penelope Leach does not take into account is that cow's milk contains six times as much casein as breast milk and it therefore produces more and larger milk curds in the stomach which are harder to digest. The end result is that the baby will not totally digest cow's milk or formula milk and is therefore excreting larger amounts so needs to take in larger volumes in the first place. She also assumes that babies are only fed five times a day at most. In a book written in 1906 about breast feeding it recommends that a six-month-old baby is fed six or seven times a day. It is best to keep breast feeding until your baby gives you the signs that milk alone is not enough. This frequently does not occur till six months or later.

WHEN TO WEAN

Nature provides babies with their first teeth at around six months and this seems the most sensible (approximate) age to start weaning.

The chewing on a crust of wholemeal bread, piece of cucumber or raw carrot will help the other teeth to come through. Another pointer for when to wean is if your baby starts feeding every two hours and this goes on for more than five days. This can indicate that he is not getting the amount of milk he needs and for some reason your supply isn't responding to the demand. Also, if a baby who had been sleeping through the night, suddenly starts waking in the night for a feed, this could be the time to introduce a small amount of solid food for his dinner. But please remember that breast is still best and that the waking could be due to other things, so only use this as a point for mixed feeding if you really cannot bear not getting enough sleep.

If your baby is a very 'sucky' baby then try not to deny him his breast and leave weaning up to him. If you start to introduce just small tastes of solid food at six months he will gradually give up the breast in conjunction with your milk drying up quite naturally. Give your baby plenty of hugs and comfort at non-feeding times so he doesn't feel the only time he is really close to you is when you are feeding him. From your point of view it is better to give up over a period of a few months as then you will be saved the pain of engorged breasts, with possible breast infections. No baby should be given any solids before four months old, as there is a high possibility that allergies will be induced due to the lack of maturity of the digestive tract. Also most of the food will be going in one end and out of the other, again due to lack of maturity. However, all babies should be on some solids by eight months as the risk of infection has been shown to be higher in babies fed exclusively on breast milk past this age. The baby's iron stores will also be getting low by this age, as there is some iron in breast milk but not enough to provide all the baby's needs. A premature baby may run out of iron stores earlier than a full-term baby, so ask your doctor to test a drop of her blood at least once in the first six months.

THE BABY'S FIRST FOOD

Now that we have answered the question of when, the next burning question is what? Your baby will probably only eat one or two teaspoons of food to start with as she has little idea of how to swallow solids as opposed to liquids which were nicely delivered to the back of her mouth. In her attempts to swallow, her tongue will come forward and push most of it out. Don't try to push more food on her than she wants as this will only make her gag. Also her digestive system needs to get used to processing different things, so the slower the better.

Healthy babies, as with healthy adults, need food that is fresh, unprocessed, additive-free, sugar-free (and that includes sucrose, glucose, dextrose, maltose and fructose), salt-free and low in fat. In other words food that is close to how it is found in nature. The baby will eventually be eating the food that you eat (which is of course completely healthy) so she will need to get used to eating this way right from the start. Below I have given suggestions on how to eat healthily without using lots of packaged baby foods. Packaged baby foods are improving all the time; they no longer contain artificial additives and some are sugar free (Heinz do some pure fruit purées that are just that and useful as a stand-by). However, the idea that a baby needs fibre or shouldn't have sugar on his roast beef dinner (made by Boots) has not filtered through yet. As with adult food, if you are going to use the occasional prepared food, read the label – if it contains any cereal it should be wholemeal and unrefined, it should not contain any of the sugars listed above, modified starch or hydrolyzed vegetable protein or any ingredient that you do not understand.

FIBRE FOR BABIES

Some mothers will not give their baby a high-fibre diet as it 'goes straight through them'. What they often mean is they are getting three dirty nappies a day and cannot be bothered changing them all that often. How I look at it is that I would rather change three dirty nappies a day for a year or two than nurse an older person through the horrors of bowel cancer when your 'baby' is grown up. In this day and age of disposable nappies it really isn't that bad. As with an adult a healthy bowel should be emptying itself two to three times a day and much of the food will come out as recognizable lentils or grape skins. Much of this is due to the fact that a baby cannot chew foods properly. The high-fibre revolution is getting through to babies as Farley's now produce a wholemeal rusk – it's a shame that they put sugar in it!

PREVENTING ALLERGIES

At the start of weaning give your baby food that is very easily digested and that is unlikely to cause an allergic reaction. Cooked, puréed vegetables and fruits are a good start. If a fruit or vegetable can be given raw then leave it raw, for example bananas, avocados, very ripe William's pears or paw paws. The later that you introduce a food the less likelihood there is of producing an allergic reaction. So if you suspect your child may react allergically (if there is, for instance, a family history of allergy) or you just want to be absolutely certain that your child does not have any allergies, introduce potential allergens as late as you can. Below is a list of foods and food groups with those most likely to give an allergic reaction at the bottom. So start by giving the foods at the top and as each one is cleared move down the list.

◆ Vegetables
◆ Fruits (except oranges)
◆ Nuts and seeds
◆ Pulses and beans
◆ Rice
◆ Meat
◆ Oats, barley and rye
◆ Oranges
◆ Wheat
◆ Milk products
◆ Eggs

Introduce one or two foods on each day and make a note of which foods you have given and any possible reaction. A reaction may be anything from a severe to mild eczema, excessive sleepiness, a runny nose, an ear infection, excessive thirst, over-activity or asthmatic breathing. If you notice a reaction withdraw that food and carry on with new foods once the reaction has died down. You can double check your observations a few months later when the reaction may have disappeared as the digestive system matures. The last four foods should not be introduced until nine or 10 months – this also applies to any foods that either the mother or father is known to have a reaction to.

BABY-FOOD PUREES

Your newly weaned baby will still be getting a large amount of nourishment from breast milk and you may well find that you are breast feeding as much as before. This is quite all right, in fact it is to be encouraged that you breast feed a large amount right up to the age of one. Assuming your baby is getting most of his protein, fat and carbohydrate from milk, you would be best to feed him plenty of vitamin and mineral-rich vegetables and fruit. These are very easy to prepare – just cook a combination of vegetables or fruit, and there is no need to add sugar, and purée in a liquidizer, food processor, mouli or special baby-food blender. Here are some good combinations:

- Carrots – alone
- Cauliflower and turnip
- Carrots, spinach and cauliflower
- Broad beans and cauliflower or carrot and a very little celery
- Jerusalem artichokes and carrot
- Peeled courgettes (the skins can be bitter) and fennel
- Leek and potato
- Swede, turnip and potato

But do experiment yourself. There is no limit to the number of combinations you can come up with. To save time and effort, not to mention disappointment at your baby rejecting your lovingly prepared purées, you can freeze these mixtures. Start by using ice-cube trays for the tiniest amounts (you can also express breast milk and freeze in sterilized ice-cube trays to make food taste more like what baby's used to) and progress onto small jars and yoghurt pots with lids.

As time goes on you can slowly add other ingredients to these basic vegetable purées. Try adding red split lentils, cooked bean sprouts, well-cooked brown rice, black-eyed beans and other pulses, milk, cheese, yoghurt or soya milk. You may find your baby doesn't immediately take to some of these flavours. If this is so leave it out and try again in two weeks' time. (See Chapter 15 for more information.)

Breakfasts can be more puréed vegetables. They do not have to be sweet cereals or fruit. This is an unnecessary way to educate a sweet tooth from a very early age. As you introduce cereals into the diet more, you can cook brown rice flour as you would semolina and add puréed fruit for a lovely breakfast. An easier alternative is to pour boiling water on three teaspoons of fine oatmeal and leave to stand for a few minutes. Puréed fruit, mashed banana, yoghurt, expressed breast or cow's milk may be added to this. Millet flakes may be bought in health food shops and these can be prepared in the same way as for oatmeal. As the child gets older, porridge oats may be used in place of oatmeal and the banana may be sliced instead of mashed.

HEALTHY BABY SNACKS

It will be many years before your child will be able to survive a full day without any 'in-between meal' snacks. To start with you will probably find the following pattern will fit his needs:

on waking	:	breast milk
1–2 hours later	:	breakfast
1–3 hours later	:	breast milk
mid-day	:	lunch
during afternoon	:	breast milk
early evening	:	dinner
followed by	:	breast milk and BED

You notice that I have been purposefully vague about the times at which all these events happen. This is so you can fit the schedule into your own baby's waking and sleeping patterns. This is only a guideline to show you how to feed a baby every two to three hours and remain sane. You will also notice how this apparently weaned baby is still getting four breast feeds a day. He needs it and will carry on needing it until he is well into the swing of eating – maybe at 11 or 12 months. As your baby drops her breast feeds you will need to substitute other healthy snacks. They do not have to come out of bright packets and cost a fortune. Your baby is simply hungry and needs real food. A slice of wholemeal bread, rice cake, oatcake or piece of fruit will satisfy this need. By restricting the 'bright pack' kind of snack you should be educating your child not to ask for all the hundreds of snacks that are purposefully laid out at her level in the supermarket. You will also be avoiding the 'snack syndrome', when a child would rather have snacks than meals. After all, if you knew that for in-between-meal snacks you got brightly coloured packets of 'Monster Munch', chocolate biscuits or even Smarties and for lunch it was spinach, boiled egg or baked potato, wouldn't you choose to live off in-between-meal snacks?

HOW MUCH DOES MY BABY NEED?

One of the most common questions mothers ask is how much should my baby eat? While some mothers are thinking their babies are not getting enough because they are still not sleeping through the night and do not have rolls of puppy fat, others are thinking theirs are overfed because they seem to be constantly eating and still have 'chubby' thighs and face. There are a few important points to make here.

Firstly, it is very hard to underfeed a western baby if food is made available three times a day. A baby not sleeping through the night can be due to many reasons, one of which can be not getting enough food. So try for a few nights giving some extra food at the last meal of the day (do not force feed). If it makes no difference go back to your old feeding patterns. A baby or toddler will know how much food he wants. All you need to do is take out the greed element, so don't offer the dreaded snack foods including extra sweet things, bright packages or salty foods. If a child is hungry a piece of bread and butter will satisfy him. If he is greedy only a chocolate biscuit will do.

A baby's natural make-up is to have a certain amount of fat. How much depends on inherited traits, whether she is about to do a growth spurt (before a spurt she may well look a little fatter, whereas after a spurt she may well look lanky), how active she is and also how much you are feeding her. If she is obviously very much fatter than her peers then you are probably overfeeding. If so, are you giving her too many snacks, are you giving her undiluted fruit juice and no water, are you giving her too much milk to drink, is she eating very fatty foods (cheese, meat, eggs and cooking oil included), are you feeding her more than she really wants (just one more spoon to finish off the bowl)? On the other hand, if your baby has no rolls of fat and does not have a chubby face, look at the parents first to see if they are also slimly built. Secondly, ask yourself if he seems lethargic and not full of energy and is sleeping a lot. If this is the case then you are probably not feeding enough. Try to make food more available. Perhaps you are sticking too rigidly to his three meals a day. A baby needs snacks since he cannot survive the six or so hours between some meals so make sure he is getting enough protein and at least some unsaturated oil (this can be obtained from ground nuts, grains, avocado pears or vegetable oil). If you are in doubt as to whether your baby is under or over fed then ask your health visitor. Usually the worry is unfounded.

THE IMPORTANCE OF CHEWING

The strongest muscle in the body for its size is the jaw muscle. It needs plenty of exercise right from the start. So give your baby banana, whole beans, vegetables that are not puréed but just chopped, pieces of apple, pear or grapes and other foods that need a bit of work, as soon as he can handle them. Most chewing is done with molars (the teeth at the back of the mouth) and these do not appear until 12 to 24 months, so some foods will be just about impossible. However, these teeth are formed and lying in wait just beneath the gums, so your baby's jaw will be effective.

THE IMPORTANCE OF MILK FOR CALCIUM

If for any reason you are not breast feeding your baby between the ages of six months and one year it is important to provide a substitute – either cow's milk or soya milk with added dolomite powder (if you cannot get dolomite powder you will need to crush dolomite tablets) which provides calcium and magnesium, much needed for bone growth. Please see the supplements chapter for the correct dosage.

There is evidence that some children who react allergically to cow's milk do not react to goat's milk. However, before the age of two years a child should not be given unpasteurized milk. If you can find a supply of pasteurized goat's milk this is fine. If you cannot, you should first check out the milking situation. Is someone milking the goat by hand into an open bucket (also open to goat hair, dung and any bacteria you care to mention) or is a proper milking machine being used, whether the sterile milk is going into an enclosed bucket or pipe system? If the latter is the case this is fine, but the milk should still be boiled and then cooled rapidly in a fridge by you at home. When using either bottles or feeding beakers for milk these should be cleaned very thoroughly and sterilized – bacteria just love milk and it is a perfect medium in which to multiply.

Drinks of mineral water or water filtered in a Brita water filter or fruit juice diluted with four parts water to one part juice will also need to be made available. Your baby will soon tell you when he is thirsty.

RECIPES FOR A HEALTHY BABY

Here are some recipes and ideas to help you on the way to feeding your baby until he is able to join in with the family meals:

——————————— Breakfast ———————————
Oatmeal or millet soaked in a little boiling water with milk, soya milk or yoghurt and banana or puréed apple or fresh, soft pear.

Brown rice flour cooked as for semolina served on its own or with the above fruit.

Snacks

Rice cakes, plain or spread with a very thin layer of peanut butter, sesame spread, sugar-free jam or sugar-free pear and apple spread. Wholemeal bread, again plain or spread with any of the above. Oatcakes as above. These usually contain salt which should not be given to a baby under nine months, so either make your own, omitting the salt, or give in small quantities to older babies. A few grapes or strawberries, pieces of apple, banana or pear.

Lunch or Dinner

CAULIFLOWER CHEESE: cook cauliflower until it is only just soft, make a cheese sauce in the usual way, with either cow's or soya milk, liquidize or mash depending on how well your baby can chew.

LENTIL SOUP: put one cup of red split lentils in two cups of cold water, add a finely chopped onion and ½ tsp Vecon (due to the salt content Vecon should not be given to babies under nine months), bring to the boil and simmer gently until lentils go to a mush, about 25 minutes.

Whole Earth or Waitrose baked beans for babies over nine months – these two brands are sugar-free.

WHOLEMEAL SPAGHETTI WITH TOMATO AND COTTAGE CHEESE SAUCE: cook wholemeal spaghetti in usual way, chop three tomatoes and half an onion, cover with water in a small pan with ½ tsp basil and simmer until soft, about 10 minutes. For small babies liquidize sauce with spaghetti and cottage cheese (use tofu – soya bean curd in place of cottage cheese if liked). For older babies just chop spaghetti and mix with tomato sauce and cottage cheese or tofu.

RAW CARROT SOUP: this is an excellent way to give raw vegetables to a small baby. Chop 8 oz raw carrots and purée in the food processor, add 2 oz ground almonds, ¼ pint sugar-free soya milk and ½ tsp mixed herbs, purée together and serve either slightly warm or cold.

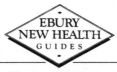

CHAPTER 14

CRYING, SLEEPING AND HYPERACTIVITY

Oﬀ all the distraught young mothers that I see the vast majority seek help because their child doesn't sleep, won't stop crying or is overly active and aggressive. Any one of these is enough to wear down the resolve of even the strongest mother. But what causes these problems and what can be done?

HYPERACTIVITY – THE NUTRITION CONNECTION

From Dr Spock to Penelope Leach hyperactivity is called a 'psycho-social problem'. And this may be part of the truth, but it is certainly not the whole truth. In recent years chemical sensitivity, food allergy, undernutrition and toxic metals have all been linked with the tell-tale signs of hyperactivity. But what exactly is hyperactivity?

In a way, the label 'hyperactive' is wrong. Many children are incredibly active and this can be a good sign of intelligence and natural curiosity, even if it leaves the mum exhausted. But a hyperactive child is quite different. Classically they are disorganized and have difficulty concentrating. Attention span is very short, often only a few seconds, so they change what they're doing all the time. Their mood is equally changeable.

'He's really such a nice child but sometimes he becomes so aggressive, literally biting or hitting me.' This sort of statement describes the rapid mood swings so often seen in hyperactive children. Their sleep is often disturbed and the child may also cry a lot. These signs may occur from birth, and before, according to a recent survey which found that excessive 'foetal kicking' during pregnancy is associated with high risk for hyperactive symptoms. But what role does nutrition play?

FOOD ADDITIVES

At least 15 years ago Dr Ben Feingold started treating hyperactive children with the Feingold diet. This is free from all artificial colours, flavourings and naturally occurring salicylates. His records and reputation speak for themselves, yet only in the past five years have his ideas begun to filter through to the medical journals. One of the first clear results came from Dr Swanson in 1980, working in Canada. He found that hyperactive children, when given a diet free of artificial food colourings, improved their behaviour. When the food dyes were then given for five days (compared to placebo) there was a measurable worsening in the children's behaviour. Children not labelled as hyperactive had no change in behaviour with the food dye diet. At exactly the same time some researchers in New York and California studied 22 children on and off food colourings. They found that only one of the children reacted badly. But her reactions were very pronounced. She was intermittently given dummy substances or a blend of seven artificial colours. Five out of seven times that the colourings were given, her behaviour changed dramatically. Over the 77 days of the trial her mother was correct in identifying five of the times the colourings were given.

Five years later, researchers at Great Ormond Street Hospital in London confirmed the diet connection. They found thhat the preservative, benzoic acid (E210), and the yellow colouring, tartrazine (E102), have the strongest effect. But these were not the only dietary offenders. In fact, 46 out of 76 children also reacted to other substances ranging from wheat to eggs.

FOOD ALLERGY AND SUGAR

The idea that foods can cause behavioural changes is nothing new, although 'brain allergy' is still not accepted by the medical profession at large. For example, wheat gluten sensitivity is found in four per cent of all schizophrenic patients, according to the Brain Bio Center. Sometimes children and adults react badly to all grains (oats, rye, barley), milk produce, eggs, oranges and many other foods. Often sugar is implicated, although this may not be strictly an allergic reaction. Sugar is a stimulant and can cause rapid changes in blood sugar levels. This factor alone can cause changes in behaviour and doesn't necessarily mean allergy.

It's also known that some foods that aren't stimulants cause their allergic symptoms by causing low blood sugar levels. Often hypoglycaemia and allergy are confused. But sugar sensitivity is probably not a common cause of hyperactivity. Dr Gross in Illinois, USA, studied 51 hyperactive children. Only one showed a consistent adverse reaction to sugar, which he thought was due to sucrose deficiency, which is the enzyme that helps break sugar down. Other researchers have found a stronger link between behaviour and sugar. For example, a prison study in Virginia lowered the sugar intake of a group of juvenile delinquents. Analysis of 934 infractions committed by the 276 juveniles over a two-year period showed an 82 per cent lower incidence of assault in those on the low sugar diet. Research at the Massachusetts Institute of Technology found that the higher the proportion of refined carbohydrates, the lower the IQ. The difference was a staggering 25 IQ points!

HEAVY METALS

Lead and cadmium are the two most important toxic minerals known to induce hyperactivity by interfering with nerve transmission. All emotions and thinking processes as well as activity levels and the experience of pain are determined by the state of the nervous system. So too is the rate of development. Although most brain cells are already developed at birth, from then on a massive 'wiring' job takes place, cross-linking nerve cells, building bridges of communication. In fact, each nerve cell makes somewhere in the region of 10,000 connections – that is unless there's lead around. Then only 9,000 connections are made. It's not a difficult step to see how these minerals can easily affect your child's behaviour. Lead and cadmium make the nerve cells 'fire' too much, causing hyperactivity and over-sensitivity to hunger and pain. Children with high lead levels may not sleep so well, and demand constant attention.

Another mineral that may be involved is copper. Copper acts as a stimulant to the brain, and excess copper may be a factor in hyperactivity.

The mineral zinc, on the other hand, has a protective and beneficial effect. Babies whose mother's zinc status is high are larger at birth, have a bigger head circumference, and a particularly low risk for mental retardation. But, perhaps most important of all, zinc helps to combat the dangerous effects of lead and cadmium.

Calcium and magnesium are also vital for nerve transmission and balanced moods. Not only are they the main constituents of bones and teeth but they are also involved in a push-me-pull-you effect in nerves and muscles, acting as natural tranquillizers. Muscles work through a series of contractions and relaxations which are governed by the levels of calcium and magnesium in and around the muscle cell. These two are also vital for nerve function and it is lead's interference with calcium in the nerve cell that causes the behavioural and intellectual impairment associated with lead. While most people know that calcium is high in milk produce, unfortunately milk is a very poor source of magnesium. Nuts and seeds, especially sesame and sunflower seeds, are the highest sources of calcium and magnesium. These can be ground and fed to the baby once on solids – and, of course, breast-feeding mums. Green leafy vegetables are also rich in these minerals.

THE OPTIMUM NUTRITION APPROACH

As well as determining allergies and testing for toxic metal levels the 'optimum nutrition' approach of correcting vitamin and mineral deficiencies and ensuring a healthy diet is often needed to get good results. Also, the essential fatty acid, gamma-linolenic acid, has been shown to help lessen allergic reactions, which are often unavoidable when children go to stay with friends or go to parties. However, researchers simply using megadoses of vitamins (like 1 to 3 g of B3 and up to 1 g of B5 in children!) have shown mixed results. The use of such large amounts of vitamins without first determining the likelihood of deficiency is a dubious way of assessing the importance of nutrition in hyperactivity.

As you can see, hyperactivity, crying and poor sleeping patterns can be caused by a number of environmental factors. It is often not easy to treat these problems and it is usually best to explore the possibilities with a qualified nutritionist.

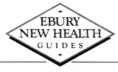

CHAPTER 15

FOOD FADS AND FUSSINESS

'My child will only eat chocolate yoghurt.' 'My child will only eat spaghetti hoops and baked beans.' 'My child will only eat potatoes, carrots and baked beans.' Anyone who has anything to do with children will recognize these phrases well and there are five points to remember in these situations:

1 Provided the diet is balanced young children don't need great variety. While they do prefer sweeter vegetables like carrots to bitter foods they do not have great taste discrimination. Texture is more important to them.

2 If you do not have chocolate yoghurt, spaghetti hoops or whatever other junk food these children decide to eat, then you will never get into this situation as the option isn't there.

3 Ensure that your child has adequate zinc status and is therefore able to taste to his full capacity.

4 From the very start, eating should be a matter of satisfying appetite, not something you do for mummy or something you do tidily or even for starving people. Eating should be an independent thing that the child does for himself as soon as possible using spoon or hands, whichever is easier – and preferably messier.

5 For a small baby texture is usually more important than flavour so be careful to purée properly and try to avoid slimy things altogether.

PREVENTION IS BETTER THAN CURE

As it is well known that prevention is better than cure, this is the easiest way to tackle the problem. The majority of food fads arrive out of emotions, getting attention or upsetting mum. The fewer emotions that are around at meal time the better. Try not to give out lashings of praise for an empty bowl, and try not to appear too hurt when you have to throw away your lovingly prepared vegetable casserole, puréed to just the right consistency. If your child wants more soup, give it to him; he may be extra hungry today due to an impending growth spurt, cold or just lots of toddler activity. It is equally important not to withhold food as it is not to push it upon an unwilling toddler — let *his* appetite lead his eating, not *your* dogmas. If your baby takes a temporary dislike to something, don't push it; it is far better to have two weeks without eggs than a whole lifetime. Just reintroduce the food again after a short period and see what happens.

GIVE THEM CHOICES

It will be a long time before a child has the complete capability to make a choice between, say, baked beans and spaghetti. A toddler will not understand if you say 'What do you want for lunch today?' Whereas if you hold up a banana and a pear and say 'Do you want a banana or a pear?' he may understand and state his preference. You need to decide how much your child can understand and in any unsure situation step in with a suggestion. Your child needs your understanding and authority. Don't give your toddler too much choice, as he will not know what to do with it. It is far better to lay out the family lunch table with two or three different choices of things your toddler can eat, than to offer him the whole larder. If he doesn't want what is offered, assume he is not hungry. Don't carry on offering him more and more choice – this is one sure route to fussiness.

REWARDS AND SNACKS

In the previous two chapters are guidelines to prevent your child becoming a snack eater. Do not give interesting foods as snacks. If a toddler is really hungry in between meals she will happily eat a piece of wholemeal bread. There are also guidelines on not rewarding your child with food as this only brings strong emotions into the whole situation.

DEALING WITH A FUSSY CHILD

First of all look at what your child is eating and ask yourself whether he is really getting a well-balanced diet, or at least one that isn't too bad. For instance, don't worry about a child that won't eat meat or eats large amounts of potatoes (a diet that consists solely of potatoes provides enough protein for an adult and enough carbohydrate and many of the right vitamins and minerals) or wants to live off a diet of baked beans, carrots and peas. If necessary write a food diary of exactly what is being eaten – you may be surprised. If he does appear to be getting good food then DON'T WORRY.

If, however, his diet is very imbalanced, then first of all remove the chocolate yoghurt from the house and wait – it will be a long time before your child starves! If possible, try to find a healthy alternative to the junk he craves. If it's chocolate, carob is a good alternative. It can be bought in bars or as a powder and wherever chocolate is used it can be used instead. If he craves spaghetti hoops, try substituting wholemeal spaghetti in a homemade tomato sauce.

Most important of all, pretend that you really don't care what he eats. And believe that eventually he will come round.

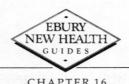

CHAPTER 16

SUGAR-FREE BABIES

CHILDREN love it. Adults crave it. Diabetes is caused by it. Teeth rot with it. But if it's so bad for us, why do we like it? The answer to this simple question provides the answer to probably a third of all western disease and the way to keep your child healthy. Let me explain.

Whether or not you like the idea, human beings belong to the family primate – monkeys and apes. And, like our ancestors, we are equipped with certain instincts – inborn programming for survival. One of these, the enjoyment of sweetness, is probably there to protect us from nature's more poisonous food. Almost anything sweet is safe. Fruits are safe, berries are safe. It's a good rule. For the plant kingdom it also makes sense, because when animals eat plants, the seeds are deposited with a pile of manure – a good start in life!

But mankind, infinitely smarter than its ancestors, learned to extract and concentrate the source of sweetness from food until in the 20th century we are left with pure, white and deadly sucrose – sugar. But why deadly? The process of refining sugar removes all the fibre, breaks down all the complex sugars (starches) and destroys most of the vitamin and mineral content. It is these very nutrients that are needed to turn sugar into energy in our bodies. So we end up without sufficient stores of the nutrients needed to process the sugar and sugar metabolism starts to go wrong.

That's half the story. The other half is all about stress. Let's start at the beginning again. All primates have a powerful system for coping with stress. It's called the fight or flight syndrome, because it's designed to help you get up a tree if you are hunted, run faster if you're hunting and heal wounds rapidly if you're fighting. Even though today's stresses are more likely to be mortgages or demands at work, the same system still operates. For example, if you're frustrated because you're stuck in a traffic jam, your blood still coagulates faster, in case you're wounded. Digestion still slows down to channel biological activity to increasing supply of sugar stores to the muscle cells for extra energy. So what has all this got do with your baby?

Sugar acts as a stressor for babies too. They also have to cope with the sudden increase in blood sugar (caused by any stress factor) by producing more and more insulin to bring the balance back to normal. If this balance is lost, both physical and mental well-being are, in turn, unbalanced. Low blood glucose (hypoglycaemia) and high blood glucose (hyperglycaemia) can have similar and wide-ranging effects: irritability, aggressive outbursts, nervousness, depression, crying spells, confusion, forgetfulness, inability to concentrate, fatigue, insomnia, headaches, palpitations, muscle cramps, excess sweating, digestive problems, allergies and excessive thirst.

It doesn't take long for the baby to learn that sugar can, at least temporarily, relieve these symptoms. Unfortunately, for most people it takes years to learn that sugar helped cause the problem in the first place. Some find out too late and end up with diabetes.

DON'T MAKE YOUR BABY A SUGAR ADDICT

But what can you do to reverse the problem and solve the addiction to sugar? The first step is not to encourage the habit in your baby. But when all is said and done how do you keep a bear away from honey? For children and adults alike the answer is first to get used to less sweet food. Sweets can be replaced with fruit or the occasional home-made fruit bar. 'Desserts' can be replaced with 'starters' or just fruit.

In fact, there's good evidence that a large part of the sweet tooth syndrome is a learned habit. This was demonstrated in a study in Israel which compared taste preferences for increasingly sweet sucrose solutions in both city and country dwellers, all 12-year-old boys. The city boys preferred a solution more than twice as sweet, and consequently had far more fillings and tooth decay. Living in Jerusalem they had more access to sweets and had clearly acquired the sugar habit (1).

MOST SUGAR IS HIDDEN

There are many different kinds of sugars, some of which occur naturally in quite high concentrations in healthy foods. Others are added. Over half our sugar intake comes from snack foods. So most of our sugar is hidden in convenience foods. Just avoiding sugar isn't enough. You also need to check the labels of the food you eat. The higher sugar is on the list of ingredients the more it contains. And sugar means dextrose, sucrose (table sugar), maltose and glucose. Two sugars which are marginally less bad are lactose (milk sugar) and fructose (fruit sugar). These do not release so rapidly into the bloodstream. So eating a lot of fresh fruit isn't a bad thing, although eating a lot of dried fruit is not so highly recommended. Honey is also concentrated sugar and is only marginally better than eating sugar. On the rare occasion when you need to add some sweetness to a dish, a little honey, molasses or maple syrup is better than sugar. Just sweetening dishes with soaked, dried fruit is better still.

HOW TO KEEP YOUR BABY SUGAR FREE

The best way to keep your baby off sugar is to go back to the natural diet and eat lots of fresh fruit. By lots, I mean lots, it would be quite all right for an 18-month-old baby to eat three bananas plus some grapes or strawberries in a day, or two soft pears and two bananas. By doing this you are getting her into the habit of eating fruit instead of cakes, biscuits and sweets.

Another good habit to encourage is drinking diluted fruit juice and plain water, or just plain water. A breast-fed baby can go from breast to juice diluted one part juice to four parts water, as well as plain bottled or filtered water. If your young child already drinks fruit juices straight, then a slow weaning process is needed, slowly diluting the juice more and more.

When weaning your baby sweetness need never come into the process. Penelope Leach suggests that when you have not made a pudding for the family you could use a commercially prepared baby dessert. But no baby needs a pudding. Nor for that matter do you. If you want to give your baby two courses for variety then why not choose the first two, i.e. a very thick lentil soup followed by vegetable purée, or vegetable soup followed by cheese and 'biscuits' (rice or oatcake or wholemeal bread). This way you are providing a meal with protein, fat and plenty of slow-releasing carbohydrate along with vitamins and minerals and plenty of taste experiences.

Up to the age of two the most likely place that she will come into contact with sugar is at coffee mornings and on social visits to friends and relatives. It is here that you will have to be strong in your convictions about not giving your child any sugar. Start by always carrying an alternative snack around with you. This can be a rice cake, wholemeal roll, oatcake, banana or a few grapes. It will be many months before she realizes that she is eating something different and possibly not as nice as everyone else, but by then she will be so used to eating fruits and bread as snacks, she may well carry on in this way. When someone asks you where your baby gets her energy from (due to the old myth that sugar equals energy) reply with a list of her day's menu – porridge, yogurt, banana, rice cake, vegetable casserole, egg, red kidney bean stew, pears and tomatoes – each one of these will be providing your baby with energy.

DON'T USE SWEETS FOR TREATS

Sugar addiction has two elements: the body's physical reaction and dependence on it and the psychological 'have a sweet – make it better' syndrome. Just as with training your child to like savoury foods it is most important to work on the psychological element from an early age. The golden rule here is: *Never give sweets, biscuits, cake or fruit as a reward for being good, as something to cheer him up either after a physical bump or because he is just miserable or bored.*

There are many adults who still have to have a piece of chocolate when they are depressed, which just goes to show that what you do for your one-year-old baby will last a lifetime. Think of yourself in the same situation as your child. If you have hurt yourself physically what you would want is attention and sympathy – not a chocolate biscuit! If your child falls down, pick him up and hold him so he feels secure. He has temporarily lost his sense of the world being a safe place, so you need to return that sense of safety with your physical strength and warmth. If the injury is at all serious your baby may be slightly shocked, which causes the release of adrenalin, causing the body to focus its energy into healing the wound. The blood will clot faster to seal the wound, and the immune system will be activated to fight off any bacteria in the cut. Digestion also shuts down, so eating is the last thing your baby should do. This is graphically illustrated by a story about a little girl who knocked a tooth out shortly after breakfast. She then spent a traumatic day with dentists nursing her injury, and was sick in the early evening. She brought back her breakfast just as it had looked in her bowl, totally undigested!

DON'T USE FOOD TO FIGHT BOREDOM

If a child is bored, one way of occupying her would be with food, but she would much prefer a trip to the local park, or a game with you. One of the most boring things for a toddler is shopping, the temptation to eat made all the stronger by continually passing food – particularly brightly coloured sweet packets placed at toddler level. Try to involve your toddler in the shopping – take a little basket with you for her to put the odd thing in. In regularly used shops she may get to know where the brown rice is and be able to fetch it for you. If your child is not up to this or the shop is totally unknown then take some toys or picture books with you. A pull-along toy would be good with lots of long shop aisles to go down and the noise needn't be too irritating for you as it is drowned out by the shop noise. The other option is to leave the child with a neighbour or relative while you shop in peace.

REWARDS

When it comes to rewards, again, put yourself in his position – would you rather have a piece of cake or a nice, loving cuddle with your baby? Up to the age of about two he still loves mum more than anything in the whole world. So if he's been good, praise him and give him a congratulatory kiss; to be accepted by you and acknowledged as a good boy by you is very important to him. If later on you find this is just not enough, you needn't use sugar; there are plenty of healthy savoury or sugar-free snacks available from health food shops, or a small toy or book.

HEALTHY SWEETS AND PUDDINGS

The need for eating sweet things is bound to arise at some point – people coming to lunch will expect a pudding, a child will come who is used to having sweets and sugar, or there will be the occasional time when even you want a sweet pudding. Here are some ideas for snacks, sweets and puddings using dried or fresh fruit and the occasional small amount of honey as a sweetener.

APRICOT DREAM

You can serve this dessert in individual glasses and decorate with fresh fruit, almonds or dried apricots. The following recipe is a variation on this, using fresh fruit in place of dried.

8 oz (225 g) apricots
¼ tsp natural vanilla essence
8 fl oz (200 g) natural yoghurt
8 oz (225 g) Quark or low-fat curd cheese
2 egg whites

1 Stew apricots in water until soft.
2 Liquidize with vanilla essence, yoghurt and curd cheese.
3 Whisk egg whites stiffly and fold into apricot mixture.
4 Cool in fridge before serving.

FRUIT FOOL

Try different combinations of fruit to ring the changes with this recipe; strawberries and/or raspberries, stewed rhubarb, stewed gooseberries or 1 part blackcurrants to 2 parts stewed apple. You may need a little honey with some of the sourer fruits.

*1 lb (450 g) fresh or frozen
    fruit
8 oz (225 g) Quark or low–fat
    curd cheese
½ tsp natural vanilla essence
2 oz (50 g) ground almonds
1 egg white, whisked stiffly*

1 Blend all ingredients, except egg white, in a liquidizer.
2 Fold in egg white.
3 Serve decorated with fruit and nuts.

RICE PUDDING

*4 oz (100 g) brown rice
2 oz (50 g) raisins
1½ pints (900 ml) milk
1 tbsp honey
grated nutmeg*

1 Put rice, raisins, milk and honey in an ovenproof dish.
2 Stir until honey is completely dissolved.
3 Sprinkle liberally with grated nutmeg.
4 Bake in an oven 300° F (150° C) gas mark 2 for 2 hours.

RASPBERRY SORBET

*1 lb (450g) raspberries
2 bananas, chopped into ½
    inch lengths*

1 Freeze whole raspberries and chopped banana.
2 Liquidize or process in a food processor and serve immediately.

The following recipes are for delicious fruit bars. These make an excellent alternative to sweets for the child who already has sweets or, on that special occasion at Christmas or parties (your friends' sweet-eating children will probably love them – particularly if you wrap them up in pretty paper or mould them into animal shapes).

DATE DELIGHT

5 oz (125 g) almonds
5 oz (125 g) rolled oats
9 oz (250 g) dried dates
  (check all stones are
  removed)
4 tbs water or orange juice
desiccated coconut,
  (optional)

Combine all the dry ingredients in a food processor and process until thoroughly chopped. Then slowly add the water or juice until it forms a ball. You may need more or less than indicated. Roll out on a board (dust with desiccated coconut if too sticky) and cut into strips, animal shapes or the letters of your child's name. If you really want a mess let your child mould his own animal shapes. Below I have given some other combinations of dried fruit and nuts.

AMAZIN' RAISIN

5 oz (125 g) almonds
5 oz (125 g) dried apple rings
5 oz (125 g) raisins
4 tbs water
½ tsp ground cinnamon
5 oz (125 g) oats

APRICOT AND ALMOND BAR

5 oz (125 g) almonds
5 oz (125 g) rolled oats
9 oz (250 g) dried apricots
4 tbs water

If you do not have the time or equipment to do these recipes there are a large number of different sugar-free bars available from health food shops, although labels still need to be read even in a health food shop as many still have large amounts of unnecessary sugar. Shepherd Boy do a very good range of sugar-free fruit bars.

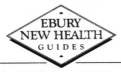

CHAPTER 17

THE ART OF CHEMICAL SELF-DEFENCE

IN the last ten years over 3,000 foods and chemicals have been added into the food we eat. Some have taken the place of natural foods, decreasing the amount of meat in a hamburger to under 30 per cent. Others are added to foods to make them look better, taste better and last longer. These are preservatives and additives. So common is the use of food additives that each one of us inadvertently eats no less than 14 lb of these chemicals each year. But are these 'permitted' additives really safe for us and our babies?

Sophie, aged two, was one of 20 children chosen to take part in a test for sensitivity to food colourings. For six months she was strictly kept away from any foods with colourings or salicylates (which are also found in aspirin, cherries and plums). Then, without her or her mother knowing what was being added, Dr Weiss added on some days dummy substances, and other days small amounts of food colourings most commonly added to our foods. Whenever the food colourings were added Sophie changed . . . like Jekyll and Hyde. She started throwing and breaking things, whining and running away and was clearly unwell. On these occasions her mother guessed she'd been given colourings. In fact, over 77 days she was given colourings six times. Her mother guessed right five times. When the daily dose was increased, 17 out of 20 children showed the same changes in behaviour.

These results alerted mothers and doctors to the problems of food additives, but no action was taken to restrict the colouring agents or even publicize the facts. Now, five years later, researchers from the Institute for Child Health and the Hospital for Sick Children in London have confirmed these results. They studied 76 'overactive' children. 62 improved on a diet free from additives. 48 different foods were found to cause a reaction and artificial colourings and preservatives were found to be the commonest provoking substances.

No action is being taken by the food industry. It's up to mothers to develop the art of chemical self-defence. Potentially harmful food additives are in many children's and baby foods. Take crisps, for example. The first ones our nutritionist, Yvonne Meek, looked at were Smiths and this is what she found. 'The ingredients list . . . antioxidants E320, E321. Looking them up in *E for Additives*, a useful guide to what's in food, these are listed as "not permitted in foods intended for babies or children". Perhaps children's most popular snack should have an "adults only" label!

'Other crisps we looked at weren't much better, except Golden Wonder ready salted plain variety, which are free of preservatives. But wotsit got in Wotsits? Lots – but top of the pops has to be Monster Munch. These have nine additives, seven of which are on the "not permitted" or "not advised" lists for children. Monsters indeed. But munch? I wouldn't if I were you!'

The worst food we could find topped the charts with no less than 20 additives! See if you can guess what it is from the ingredients list. They are: sugar, starch, salt, hydrogenated vegetable oil, whey powder, lactose, caseinate, gelling agents (E410, E407, E340), potassium chloride, adipic acid, acidity regulator (E336), stabilizer (E446), artificial sweetener (sodium saccharin), colours (E102, E110, E132, E123, E160A), flavourings, emulsifiers (E477, E322), preservative (E202), and antioxidant (E320). In case you hadn't guessed, this is a popular brand of 'banana and tropical fruit flavoured trifle'!

The introduction of E numbers, with a little guidance, will make the art of chemical self-defence much easier. In line with EEC regulations, all food additives will be allocated an E number. For the manufacturers, this means they won't have to put long lists of chemical-sounding ingredients on their products . . . just long lists of E numbers, if they choose to use them. For us members of the public at last we'll know what's in the food we buy. No longer will we be fobbed off with the all-embracing 'contains permitted additives and preservatives'.

So how do we break the E numbers code? First of all, different types of additives form different E number series: for example, colouring agents are numbered between E100 and E180. Here are the rest:

Colours	*E100*	*to*	*E180*
Preservatives	*E200*	*to*	*E290*
Anti-oxidants	*E300*	*to*	*E321*
Emulsifiers	*E322*	*to*	*E494*
Sweeteners	*E420*	*to*	*E421*
Mineral hydrocarbons	*E905*	*to*	*E907*
Modified starches	*E1400*	*to*	*E1442*

But do we really need any of these? Let's concern ourselves with the first four categories. Colours are added to make our food look good. Of course, if you don't mind eating peas that don't glow in the dark and can accept that haddock isn't naturally bright yellow, then it is better to avoid all food colourings. Except two. E101 is vitamin B2. And E160 is vitamin A. These colouring agents are actually good for you.

Preservatives prevent the growth of micro-organisms like mould. Often the effects of mould are far worse than the effects of preservatives. However, if you can buy food fresh that's the best. It's a matter of choice. Sausages, for example, contain nitrates (E250-E252) to prevent some very dangerous micro-organisms. But the more nitrates you eat the more you risk forming nitrosamines, which are potent cancer-producing chemicals. No preservatives are actually good for you.

Anti-oxidants stop food becoming rancid. This is most important for fats and oils. Nature equips foods with anti-oxidants. Seeds, high in oils, are also high in vitamin E. Vitamin E is a good anti-oxidant. Its E numbers are E306, E307, E308 and E309. Another natural anti-oxidant is vitamin C. Its E numbers are E300, E301, E302, E303 and E304. Other anti-oxidants like BHA (E320) and BHT (E321) are of dubious safety.

Emulsifiers help to bind and emulsify sauces. It's the lecithin in egg that makes mayonnaise what it is. Lecithin is E322. Other emulsifiers, like the polyphosphates, E450, are there so that more water can be added to meats, increasing the manufacturer's profits.

ADDITIVES – GOOD AND BAD

COLOURS (E100–E180)

Good	Bad	
E101 Riboflavin	E102	Tartrazine
E160 Carotene	E104–E142	Mainly coal tar or azo dyes
	E150	Caramel
	E151–E155	Coal tar dyes
	E173	Aluminium
	E174	Silver

PRESERVATIVES (E200–E290)

Good	Bad	
	E200–E203	Sorbates
	E210–E219	Benzoates
	E220–E227	Sulphur/Sulphites
	E230–E249	Misc.
	E250–E252	Nitrates
	E262	Diacetate
	E281–E283	Propionates
	E290	Carbon dioxide

ANTI-OXIDANTS (E300–E321)

Good		Bad	
E300–E304	Ascorbates	E310–E312	Gallates
E306–E309	Tocopherols	E320	BHA
		E321	BHT

EMULSIFIERS, STABILIZERS AND OTHERS (E322–E925)

Good		Bad	
E322	Lecithin	E385	EDTA
E375	Nicotinic acid	E407	Carrageenan
E440	Pectin	E513	Sulphuric acid
		E525	Potassium hydroxide
		E535	Sodium ferrocyanide
		E541	Sodium aluminium phosphate
		E631	Sodium inositate
		E635	Sodium ribonucleotide
		E905	Mineral hydrocarbons
		E924	Potassium bromate
		E925	Chlorine

To help you choose the right foods for yourself and your baby we compiled a list of the good and the bad from each section of food additives. Armed with this list our advice is to feel good about the 'goods', actively avoid the 'bads' and cut down on the rest.

If you suspect your child may be chemically sensitive you can get professional help from the Hyperactive Children's Support Group.

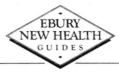

CHAPTER 18

THE PROTEIN
MYTH

A growing child needs more protein than an adult. Protein is used not for energy but for building body cells. But does this protein have to come from meat? Can a baby brought up on vegetarian foods be just as well nourished?

ANIMAL OR VEGETABLE?

Over 1.5 million people in Britain are vegetarian, eating no meat and fish, and a further 1.5 million people avoid all red meat. Vegetarianism itself is nothing new. Even the Greek mathematician Pythagoras was vegetarian. He reasoned, somewhat tangentially, that instead of offering animal sacrifices to the gods, he could offer his mathematical equations. And like his equations, he believed in keeping his diet and body in equilibrium. A recent survey by Dr Lockie and researchers at the University of Surrey has performed slightly different equations on the diets of vegans (eating no animal produce), ovo-lacto-vegetarians (eating dairy products and eggs), and wholefood omnivores (80 per cent of the diet from vegetables, cereals and wholegrains) compared to the average omnivore.

Vegan diets came closest to matching the NACNE standards for a healthy diet. However, their diets did confirm previously reported deficiencies in B2, B12 and vitamin D vitamins, all vitally important in pregnancy and lactation. Ovo-lacto-vegetarians had too much fat in their diet; however, they did have low blood levels of cholesterol, thought to be due to their high fibre intake which can lower cholesterol levels. The wholefood omnivores still ate too much fat and didn't get that much more fibre, while the average omnivores got too much fat and not enough folic acid. The researchers concluded 'Those people on a near vegan or vegetarian diet can more easily meet currently approved dietary goals. It may be prudent to restrict the intake of flesh foods to twice a week, which is the average intake in primitive tribes adopting the "hunter-gatherer" lifestyle.'

THE PROTEIN MYTH

Animal produce is the primary source of protein in the typical western diet. But is it the best kind? Protein, needed each day to help build and repair cells, consists of building blocks called amino acids. During digestion these separate amino acids are liberated for absorption, and then reconstituted by our bodies to make skin, hair, nails or other cells, all of which are examples of protein, which makes up 25 per cent of our bodyweight. Amino acids are like letters of the alphabet that can be rearranged to make thousands of different words, or types of protein.

Of the 22 amino acids mankind needs, eight must be supplied from the diet, since these cannot be made by the body. These are called the essential amino acids. A further two or three are best supplied from our diet, because, although they can be made from other essential amino acids, it is easier to get them from diet, leaving the essential amino acids free for building protein.

To judge the best source of protein, two factors must be considered. Firstly, whether the food contains the right proportion of the essential and semi-essential amino acids. And secondly, how much protein is supplied in each gram of the food.

Egg protein, for example, provides the right mix of amino acids, making it 94 per cent usable. Grains, on the other hand, lack the essential amino acids isoleucine and lysine which limit its usability to around 60 per cent. These amino acids are called the limiting amino acids.

Eggs provide 14 g of protein in 100 g of egg, the rest mainly being fat of one sort or another. So 100 g of egg provides 14 g of protein of which 94 per cent can be used.

COMPLEMENTARY PROTEINS

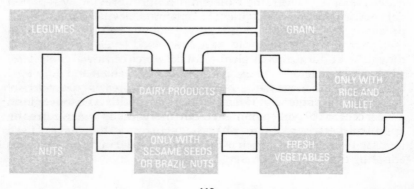

COMPLEMENTARY PROTEINS

Animal produce, gram for gram, is only a marginally better source of protein than nuts and seeds, and is no better than soya beans or milk produce. It's also a better source of fat. By combining vegetable origin foods, which complement each other's limiting amino acids, it isn't hard to get protein that is as good as meat in net usability. Only a few vegetable origin foods have such a high percentage of protein, so one would naturally need to eat more beans and rice, for example, than steak to get the same protein. But since beans and rice are high in complex carbohydrate and fibre, this is an asset not a liability. The table below shows which food groups, when combined, provide more usable protein.

PROTEIN QUANTITY VS QUALITY

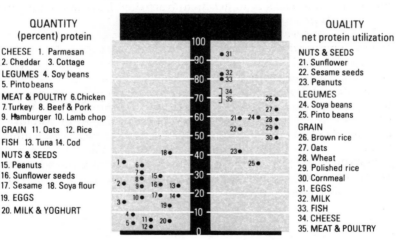

QUANTITY
(percent) protein

CHEESE 1. Parmesan
2. Cheddar 3. Cottage
LEGUMES 4. Soy beans
5. Pinto beans
MEAT & POULTRY 6.Chicken
7.Turkey 8. Beef & Pork
9. Hamburger 10. Lamb chop
GRAIN 11. Oats 12. Rice
FISH 13. Tuna 14. Cod
NUTS & SEEDS
15. Peanuts
16. Sunflower seeds
17. Sesame 18. Soya flour
19. EGGS
20. MILK & YOGHURT

QUALITY
net protein utilization

NUTS & SEEDS
21. Sunflower
22. Sesame seeds
23. Peanuts
LEGUMES
24. Soya beans
25. Pinto beans
GRAIN
26. Brown rice
27. Oats
28. Wheat
29. Polished rice
30. Cornmeal
31. EGGS
32. MILK
33. FISH
34. CHEESE
35. MEAT & POULTRY

TOO MUCH PROTEIN IS BAD FOR YOU

For the vast majority of adults and babies, getting enough protein isn't the problem. It's getting too much that creates problems. Many of us eat 50 per cent to 100 per cent more protein than we need and could cut out meat completely without lacking in protein. The 'average' 154 lb person needs 24 g of protein per day (or 0.34 g per kg of bodyweight), but my experience with several thousand patients is that, when optimally nourished with vitamins and minerals, the body becomes super-efficient and protein requirements go down. The Recommended Daily Allowance for protein is 30 per cent higher, assuming that this will provide a margin of safety for those who have particularly high needs. Professor Roger Williams and Don Davis at the University of Texas report four to tenfold variations in individuals' needs for protein. Unlike water-soluble vitamins, which are easily excreted when taken in excess, protein, which breaks down to ammonia, uric acid and urea, is toxic in large amounts and may put stress on the kidneys which eliminate these protein metabolites. Gout, for example, is one disease that results from excesses of the protein metabolite uric acid.

For babies, concentrated protein sources like eggs and meat are hard to tolerate and should not be introduced in the first nine months of life. Vegetarian sources of protein contain a higher source of complex carbohydrate and less fat and are better all round.

MICRONUTRIENTS AND THE VEGETARIAN

Another popular myth about meat is that it's the only source for many vitamins and minerals. Meat does tend to contain plenty of iron in a more available form, and also more zinc and vitamin B6. But a recent survey at the University of Carolina showed no sign of increased relative deficiency in these nutrients for vegetarians compared to meat eaters. While the bio-availability of iron in a steak is 95 per cent compared to 10 per cent for the iron in an egg, simply eating a meal high in vitamin C can increase iron absorption fourfold. A boiled egg and a glass of orange juice is a good combination.

THINK ZINC

Of greater concern for the vegetarian mother and baby is the mineral zinc. This is poorly supplied in foods of vegetable origin and, depending on where the food is grown and whether phosphate fertilizers, which prevent zinc uptake, have been used, can be deficient in the vegan diet. Since the recommended daily intake is 15 mg and the average daily intake in Britain is between 9 and 10 mg, it isn't just vegetarians that need to be concerned. In the study at the University of Carolina 30 per cent of the vegetarians and 22 per cent of the non-vegetarians were found to have low zinc status.

Vitamin B6 is also found in larger amounts in animal produce because of its role in protein metabolism. Although cooking will destroy some of the B6 it is likely that a vegetarian diet may be low in this too. So people on a diet which is high in foods of vegetarian origin need more B6 and zinc.

Fat-soluble vitamins A, D and E are also relatively high in animal produce because they can be stored. The levels will, of course, vary on the nutrition of the animal in question. However, vitamin A is well supplied in leafy vegetables, and particularly carrots and beetroot, so provided these are often eaten, the vegetarian need not fear. Vitamin D is made in the skin in the presence of sunshine and should be supplied to the young baby in milk. Vitamin E is highest in nuts and seeds.

The vitamin most associated with deficiency in the vegetarian diet is vitamin B12. However, this is only a potential problem in vegans, as milk and eggs provide plenty of B12. So do fermented soya products, spirulina, comfrey . . . and bugs. A survey on vegetarians in India identified bugs as the protective factor against B12 deficiency!

ONE MAN'S MEAT IS ANOTHER MAN'S POISON

So what's good about meat? That depends on the meat. Today's steak is very different from the meat of our ancestors. Not only has the fat percentage in meat doubled, but also the use of antibiotics and growth hormones in animal husbandry, followed by nitrates for meat preservation, has changed the very nature of what we call meat.

The increasing levels of nitrates and nitrites both in meat and vegetable produce is of growing concern. Nitrates are not dangerous in themselves, but can be converted in the plant or in the mouth and digestive tract to nitrites. These can then react with amines (protein-like substances) to produce nitrosamines – one of the most powerful carcinogens known to man. Nitrates and nitrites are added to meat products to preserve the meats. There are four forms used, potassium nitrite (E249), sodium nitrite (E250), sodium nitrate (E251) and potassium nitrate which is saltpetre (E252). They are used mainly in sausages, canned meat, pies, bacon and other cured meats.

The best forms of meat are therefore free-range chicken or game. Lamb is less likely to be treated with growth hormones and antibiotics than beef and pork. The best types of fish are deep-sea fish not exposed to polluted coastal waters. These can also be excellent sources of the essential fatty acids EPA and DHA which have a protective effect against heart disease. Freshwater fish caught in polluted waters are best avoided.

But vegetables don't escape all nasty chemicals either. In fact, more nitrates come to us from vegetables than any other source. Nitrates act as fertilizers, speeding up the plant's growth. But when too much is used, the plant simply stores the nitrates, which are passed on to us. These can then be converted to nitrites and then nitrosamines. On average, we take in 64 mg of nitrates a day from vegetables, and 92 mg a day in all. So vegetarians and meat-eaters alike, choose your vegetables carefully too.

ONE STEP AT A TIME

Unless inspired by conscience, changing to an all vegetarian diet is probably not the best way to start improving your diet. The first goal should be reduce meat eating to two or three times a week. Then it is best to stop eating red meat. Last year I set myself a target of eating meat only 12 times. This year I am a 'fishitarian', eating only fish. The same rules apply for your child. And if you follow the guidelines in this book there is no chance of your child being deficient in protein.

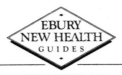

CHAPTER 19

SUPPLEMENTS FOR A HEALTHY CHILD

ACCORDING to Dr Roger Williams, often called the founder of the new nutrition, 'The greatest hope for increasing (health and) lifespan can be offered if nutrition – from the time of pre-natal development up to old age – is continuously of the highest quality.' Although diet is crucial and the right place to start, every child can benefit from the proper vitamin and mineral supplementation.

WHEN SHOULD YOU START SUPPLEMENTING?

As soon as a child has stopped receiving the majority of his nourishment from the mother's milk, supplementation should start. This preventive approach is nothing unusual. Every child can receive free of charge vitamin drops from the DHSS. Many women are not aware of this and sometimes the form filling required puts others off. For babies on formula milk these drops are designed to be taken in addition to those provided in the formula. The vitamin drops contain vitamin A 2,000 iu, vitamin D 400 iu, B1 1 mg, B2 0.4 mg, B3 0.5 mg, B6 0.5 mg and vitamin C 50 mg.

While this may provide the basic levels required for these nutrients, many other important nutrients are excluded. Especially important for the growing child are vitamin A to build up strong membranes less permeable to infection; vitamin D to aid the absorption of calcium; B vitamins and vitamin C involved in brain development; calcium and magnesium for healthy bones; zinc to maintain the integrity of RNA and DNA and assist in growth; essential fatty acids because these get incorporated into every cell – especially brain cells; and also iron, chromium, selenium and manganese.

The ideal daily intake for these nutrients is shown overleaf, compared to the Recommended Daily Allowances. The third column shows the sort of level of these nutrients that your baby will get from following the recommendations in this book. The final column shows the amounts by which even a good diet falls short.

THE IDEAL DAILY PROGRAMME

Nutrient	RDA	Optimum Level	From Optimum Diet	Minimum Supplemental Level
Vitamins				
A	900 iu	4,000 iu	15,000 iu	(4,000 iu)
D		400 iu	40 iu	400 iu
E		20 iu	5 iu	20 iu
C	20 mg	200 mg	180 mg	100 mg
B1 (thiamine)	0.5 mg	5 mg	1 mg	5 mg
B2 (riboflavin)	0.6 mg	5 mg	1 mg	5 mg
B3 (niacin)	7 mg	10 mg	7 mg	5 mg
B5 (pantothenic acid)		10 mg	4 mg	5 mg
B6 (pyridoxine)		5 mg	2 mg	5 mg
B12		5 mcg	1 mcg	2 mcg
Folic Acid		100 mcg	200 mcg	50 mcg
Biotin		150 mcg	?	50 mcg
Minerals				
Sodium		1,500 mg	868 mg	
Potassium		3,000 mg	3,200 mg	
Calcium	600 mg	600 mg	624 mg	300 mg
Magnesium		200 mg	240 mg	150 mg
Iron	7 mg	7 mg	7 mg	5 mg
Zinc		7 mg	5 mg	5 mg
Chromium		35 mcg	?	10 mcg
Manganese		1.5 mg	?	1 mg
Selenium		30 mcg	?	10 mcg

GETTING THE RIGHT SUPPLEMENTS

The major difficulty with getting the right supplements for your child is availability. Of all those we've checked only obscure American formulas, or one British manufacturer, Health + Plus, came close to providing the right levels in one tablet. Health + Plus's Children's Chewable is the best formula currently available. A one-year-old child just needs one of these tablets a day, preferably with breakfast. Supplements are better used if taken with food. Since B and C vitamins can boost energy it is best not to give them last thing at night.

ADJUSTING FOR AGE

Nutrient needs alter with age. The chart below shows the ideal intakes of each nutrient from 0 to 10. Up to age two these can be met with one Health + Plus Children's Chewable. From two to five give two and from five to 10 three a day.

OPTIMUM DAILY INTAKES FROM AGE ONE TO ELEVEN

Nutrient	Less than 1	Age 1	2	3–4	5–6	7–8	9–11
Vitamins							
A	4,000 iu	4,500	5,000	5,500	6,000	7,000	7,500
D	400 iu	400	400	400	400	400	400
E	20 iu	20	25	30	35	45	60
C	100 mg	100	200	300	400	500	600
B1 (thiamine)	5 mg	5	6	8	12	16	20
B2 (riboflavin)	5 mg	5	6	8	12	16	20
B3 (niacin)	7 mg	10	14	16	18	20	22
B5 (pantothenic acid)	10 mg	10	15	20	25	30	35
B6 (pyridoxine)	5 mg	5	7	10	12	16	20
B12	5 mcg	6	7	8	9	10	10
Folic Acid	100 mcg	100	120	140	160	180	200
Biotin	150 mcg	150	180	210	240	270	300
Minerals							
Sodium	3,000 mg	3,000	3,000	3,000	3,000	3,000	3,000
Potassium	3,000 mg	3,500	3,750	4,000	4,250	4,500	5,000
Calcium	600 mg	600	700	800	900	1,000	1,100
Magnesium	200 mg	200	225	250	300	350	375
Iron	7 mg	7	8	8	9	10	10
Zinc	7 mg	7	8	9	10	12	14
Chromium	35 mcg	35	37	40	43	45	50
Manganese	1.5 mg	2	2.5	3	3.5	4	4.5
Selenium	30 mcg	33	37	40	43	47	50

ARE THERE ANY DANGERS WITH SUPPLEMENTING CHILDREN?

Children tend to be more susceptible to vitamin toxicity than adults. As with all nutrients it is the dosage that counts. However, the doses listed above are well within any potentially toxic limits for even the most sensitive child and are therefore non-toxic.

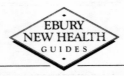

CHAPTER 20

RECIPES FOR
A HEALTHY CHILD

B Y now you will already have given your toddler a really good
nutritional start in life and you yourself will be far more confident
about feeding your child. This chapter gives guidelines for feeding the
whole family and not just the child as it is important that the whole
family eats the same healthy food, otherwise you will never be able to
keep your toddler out of the biscuit tin. Your placid baby has now
turned into a toddler and is beginning to notice exactly what is going
on around him and will want to join in with whatever you are doing,
including what you are eating.

The most important health food that you should have in great
abundance is fruit and vegetables. Nearly all children love fruit so
make sure you always have plentiful supplies.

A growing child will need a concentrated protein source and you can
select from the following: soya products such as soya milk and tofu,
milk products including yoghurt, cheese and milk, eggs, fish, chicken.
As long as your child is eating one of these direct protein sources a day
he is probably getting enough.

It goes without saying that you should not be giving your toddler
sugar, artificial additives, salt, tea or coffee. As far as the no's go the
same rules apply as for weaning. A child's kidneys may now be
mature enough to excrete salt and not produce immediate major
health problems, but there are many other reasons for not adding salt.
These include training a palate to not crave salt, not overworking the
kidneys and so preventing kidney failure in later life, and preventing
hypertension in later life. Just because the food manufacturers think
your child can now eat salt doesn't mean it's good for them! The same
goes for additives. One of the worst foods in both these respects is
potato crisps.

Here are some recipes to serve as a guideline; however, you'll do well
to purchase a good wholefood cookery book.

RECIPES AND EATING IDEAS

Here are some very practical ideas for feeding your toddler. The recipes are only a start so do use your imagination. The chewiness of the recipes varies, as between the age of 18 months and three years the number of teeth will vary quite considerably from child to child. Do not forget that even a child who hasn't cut his teeth still has them lying just under the gum and will easily demolish apple pieces if encouraged.

Breakfasts

Muesli soaked overnight in milk or soya milk served with chopped banana or apple, grated or chopped.

Low fat live yoghurt with chopped pear or banana and wheatgerm.

Porridge made in the usual way without sugar or salt with a banana or on its own (toddlers like bland food).

Boiled egg with wholemeal soldiers.

Snacks

Wholemeal bread with or without a spread such as peanut butter, sugar-free jam or a small amount of honey.

Fresh fruit.

Rice cakes, oatcakes or salt-free wholemeal crispbreads.

Quick Lunches and 'Emergency' Meals

Scrambled egg – whisk one egg with a small amount of milk, chop a tomato, put both in non-stick pan and lightly scramble in usual way.

Baked beans – use sugar and additive-free brands (Waitrose or Whole Earth).

Sandwiches – in the summer have a 'picnic' in the garden: wholemeal bread with cottage cheese and cucumber or other healthy fillings.

Raw carrot soup – fantastically nutrient rich.

Put 1 lb (450 g) chopped carrots in food processor and process until a fine purée is achieved, add 4 oz (125 g) ground almonds, ½ pint (300 ml) milk, 1 low-salt vegetable stock cube, 1 tsp mixed herbs and process until well mixed. Serve cold in summer or warm very gently. Do not over-heat.

Salad made of whatever ingredients your child will eat. Large lumps of chopped carrot will be popular with older toddlers, whereas very finely chopped cucumber, tomato, alfalfa sprouts with a little mayonnaise and yoghurt or cottage cheese will go down well with younger ones.

Lumps of cheese with apple or tomato and wholemeal bread.

Follow any of these with fresh fruit and water to drink.

Main Meal Dishes

The following recipes are to serve four adults. While it is ideal to give your toddler freshly cooked food, when time and his schedule does not allow, you can either cook in late afternoon and give the toddler his portion first or cook for an evening meal and keep his portion in the fridge for lunch the next day.

LENTIL SOUP

8 oz (225 g) brown or
  continental lentils
1¼ pints (750 ml) water
1×14 oz tin tomatoes (or
  1 lb (450 g) fresh
  tomatoes)
2 tsp oregano
1 tsp Vecon
2 cloves crushed garlic
freshly ground black pepper

Simmer lentils until tender in water in a covered pan. Add tomatoes, oregano, garlic, Vecon and pepper. Simmer for a further 5 minutes.

FARMHOUSE VEGETABLE SOUP

This is where you can really experiment with different vegetables. Try leek and potato, or cauliflower, or carrot or a combination of swede, carrot and turnip.

1½ lb (700 g) chopped fresh
  vegetables, e.g. carrots,
  leeks, potatoes, courgettes,
  tomatoes, cauliflower
1 medium onion
1 low-salt vegetable stock
  cube
2 tsp mixed herbs

Slice the onion and simmer in a little water until soft, add the chopped vegetables in combination or a single one. Add herbs and stock cube. Cover and simmer until vegetables are still slightly crunchy. Liquidize or purée.

HUMMUS

A delicious chick pea pâté that can be eaten from a very young age. Babies may like less garlic and lemon juice and more water to make it sloppier. Older children can eat it with a spoon or spread it on bread or oatcakes. You can make double quantities and freeze some.

4 oz (100 g) chick peas
1 garlic clove, crushed
1 tbsp olive oil
juice of 1 lemon
2 tbsp natural yoghurt
1 tbsp tahini
    (available from health
    food shops)

Soak the chick peas overnight, cover with fresh water and simmer for 30 minutes with the garlic or until soft. Put all ingredients in a liquidizer and purée, adding extra water if necessary.

VEGETABLE CASSEROLE

1 tbsp olive oil
2 large onions, sliced
1 lb (450 g) carrots, sliced
1 lb (450 g) potatoes, cut
    into bite-size pieces
1 medium cauliflower,
    broken into florets
8 oz (250 g) mushrooms,
    wiped and sliced
2 tbsp wholemeal flour
1 pint (600 ml) water
2 low-salt vegetable stock
    cubes
1 tbsp tomato purée
3 bay leaves
black pepper

Heat the oil in a large pan and fry onion for 5 minutes. Add the rest of the vegetables and fry for a further 4 minutes, stirring often. Sprinkle in the flour, add water, stock cubes, tomato purée, bay leaves and pepper. Transfer to an oven-proof casserole and bake for 1 hour at 190° C (375° F) gas mark 5. Remove bay leaves before serving.

FISH PIE

Buy artificial-colouring-free smoked haddock. Either ask a good fishmonger or go to Marks and Spencer.

*13 oz (325 g) combined white
   fish and smoked haddock*
½ oz (10 g) butter
1 tbsp wholemeal flour
¼ pint (150 ml) milk
5 oz (125 g) prawns
*4 oz (100 g) mushrooms,
   wiped and sliced*
2 tsp mixed herbs
freshly ground black pepper
1½ lb (750 g) potatoes
2–3 tbsp milk
2 oz (50 g) Cheddar cheese

Steam the fish in a small amount of water for 15 minutes. Meanwhile make a béchamel sauce out of the butter, flour and milk. Combine fish, sauce, prawns, mushrooms, herbs and pepper. Cook and mash the potatoes. Add the milk and freshly ground black pepper. Place the fish mixture in an oven-proof dish and top with mashed potatoes. Sprinkle with grated cheese and bake for 30 minutes at 200° C (400° F) gas mark 6.

KEDGEREE

Make to a standard recipe omitting any salt, using brown rice instead of white and, again using smoked haddock with either no colouring or a natural colouring. When cooking brown rice, it is ideal not to over-cook it, as then it turns into a simpler carbohydrate and will not keep your toddler going for so long! However, rice is not that easy to chew so you may need to cook it for longer to start with, cooking it less and less as your child grows up. The maximum time needed will be 45 minutes, the minimum, ideal time being 25 minutes.

SPAGHETTI NAPOLITANA

*12 oz (350 g) wholemeal
   spaghetti*
2 medium onions
2 tbsp olive oil
3 medium carrots
8 oz (200 g) mushrooms
1 clove garlic, crushed
1 small green pepper
4 oz (100 g) tomato purée
*2 tsp Vecon or vegetable
   stock*
2 tsp thyme

Heat the oil in a large pan and fry the sliced onion and garlic in it. Add the carrots, green pepper and mushrooms all sliced and fry for a few more minutes. Add the Vecon, thyme and tomato purée. Add water to easily cover and simmer for 20 minutes. Process briefly in a food processor or liquidizer. Meanwhile, put spaghetti in plenty of boiling water and boil for 12 minutes.

MUSHROOM AND RAISIN PILAF

A quick and easy recipe that you can leave to cook while getting on with other things.

8 oz (225 g) brown rice
½ oz (12 g) unsalted butter
1 tbsp olive oil
1 large onion, chopped
1 pint (600 ml) water
2 oz (50 g) raisins
8 oz (225 g) frozen peas
8 oz (225 g) mushrooms, sliced
1 tsp low-salt yeast extract
1 tsp finely chopped root ginger
2 tbsp chopped parsley

Fry the rice in oil and butter in a heavy frying pan over low heat until pale brown. Add onion and cook for a further 5 minutes. Add water, raisins and mushrooms, cover and simmer until the liquid is nearly absorbed and the rice still crunchy – about 15 minutes. Add frozen peas, yeast extract and ginger and cook for a further 5 to 10 minutes until all water is absorbed and rice and peas are just cooked; add more water if necessary. Serve sprinkled with chopped parsley.

STUFFED BAKED POTATOES

Always a hit with children, even children that are used to eating beefburgers and fish fingers – a good idea when friends come to visit. Stuff with cheese, fried mushrooms, cauliflower cheese or egg.

PUDDINGS AND SWEETS

The recipes given in Chapter 17 may all be used when you wish to give your children a pudding. As a general rule of thumb when making cakes and puddings, use wholemeal flour instead of white, reduce any fat that is used and sweeten with fresh bananas, different dried fruits, molasses or honey.

USEFUL ADDRESSES

Brita Water Filters make inexpensive jug water filters for reducing toxic metal content in tap water. Brita (UK) Ltd, 51 Ashley Road, Walton-on-Thames, Surrey KT12 1HG.

Foresight provides information and personal advice on the importance of pre-conceptual care and nutrition. Foresight, The Old Vicarage, Church Lane, Witley, Godalming, Surrey GU8 5PN.

Habit Breakers run an eight-evening course that has the highest proven success in helping people to stop smoking. Habit Breakers, 18 Percy Street, London W1.

Health + Plus Vitamin Company produce good quality vitamin supplements available by mail order. Health + Plus, 118 Station Road, Chinnor, OX9 4EZ (Tel: 0844-52098).

Hyperactive Children's Support Group offer help and advice for the families of hyperactive children. HACSG, c/o Mrs I. Colquhoun, Mayfield House, Yapton Road, Barnham, W Sussex PO22 0BJ.

Institute for Optimum Nutrition has a countrywide network of nutritionists able to offer personal advice for mothers-to-be. ION, directed by the author, also runs a number of short and home study courses in optimum nutrition. ION, 3 Jerdan Place, London SW6 1BE (Tel: 01-385 7984).

La Leche League supplies mother-to-mother support on breast feeding. La Leche League of GB, BM 3424, London WC1.

National Childbirth Trust has a national network of teachers to provide ante-natal preparation, post-natal support and advice on breast feeding. National Childbirth Trust, 9 Queensborough Terrace, London W2.

Westminster Advisory Centre on Alcoholism has a number of centres in London and the South East to help people both from a psychological and nutritional level to solve their drinking problems. Westminster Advisory Centre for Alcohol, 38 Ebury St, London SW1.

**This book is to be returned on or before
the last date stamped below.**

28 SEP 1987
2 5 APR 1988
21 FEB 1990
22 . 3 . 90
-5 JUN 1990
18. NOV. 1992
-5. FEB. 1996

HOLFORD, Liz and
HOLFORD, Patrick